CKD STAGE 3 AND DIABETES TYPE 2 COOKBOOK

50 Delicious Diabetic Renal Friendly Recipes to Manage Chronic Kidney Disease and Blood Sugar Levels

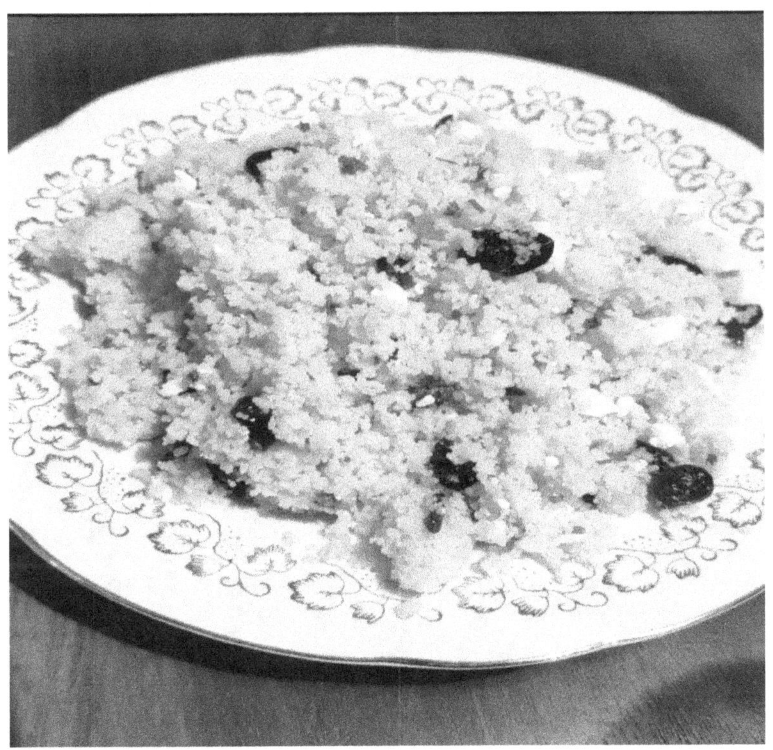

DR. COLE HULL

COPYRIGHT

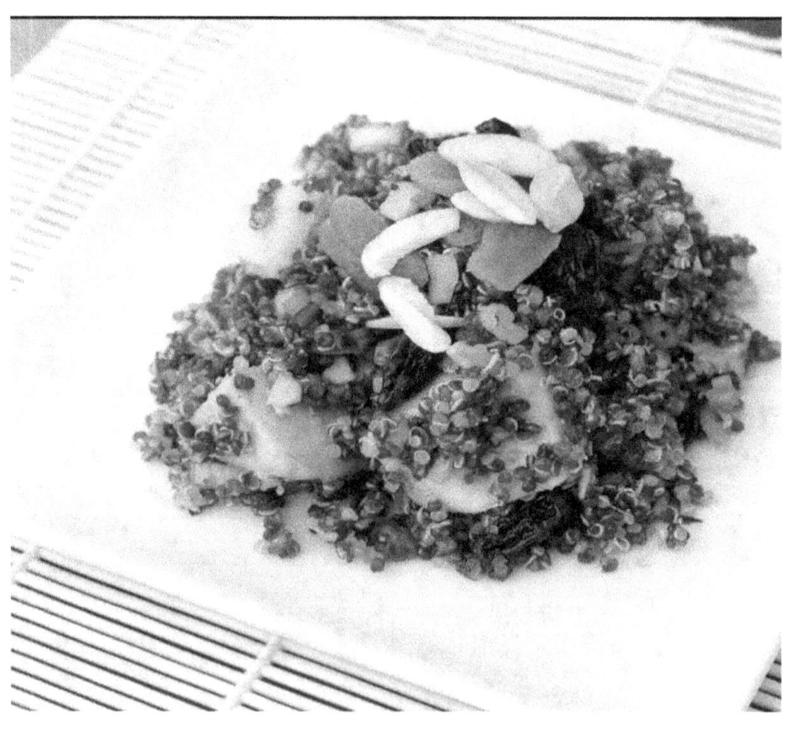

TABLE OF CONTENT

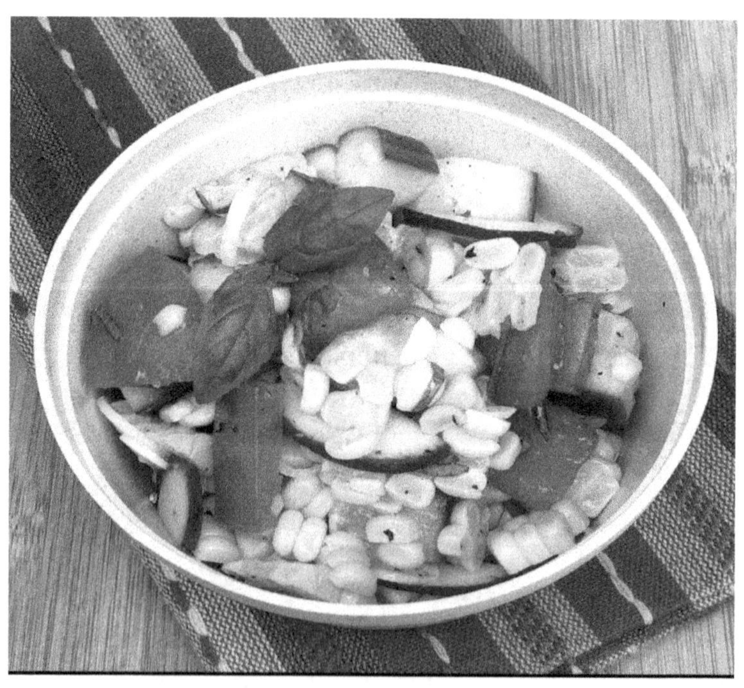

INTRODUCTION

Chronic Kidney Disease (CKD) Stage 3 and Type 2 Diabetes are both significant health conditions that require careful management, especially when it comes to diet.

For CKD Stage 3, it's important to manage protein intake, as excessive protein can put additional strain on the kidneys. A diet low in sodium, potassium, and phosphorus is also recommended to help manage blood pressure and prevent further kidney damage.

For Type 2 Diabetes, the focus is on managing blood sugar levels. This typically involves a diet that is low in simple sugars and refined carbohydrates, and high in fiber, lean proteins, and healthy fats. Monitoring carbohydrate intake and using the glycemic index to choose foods that have a lower impact on blood sugar levels can be helpful.

When managing both conditions, it's important to work closely with healthcare professionals, including a dietitian, to develop a personalized eating plan that addresses the needs of both conditions without compromising overall nutrition.

Understanding CKD Stage 3 and Diabetes Type 2

Chronic Kidney Disease (CKD) and Diabetes Type 2 are two closely related health conditions that often occur together. CKD is a progressive condition characterized by a gradual loss of kidney function over time. Stage 3 CKD is a moderate form of the disease, where the kidneys are still functioning but not as efficiently as they should. Symptoms may be mild or non-existent, making it crucial to manage the condition proactively to prevent further progression.

Diabetes Type 2, on the other hand, is a metabolic disorder that affects the way your body processes blood sugar (glucose). It's often linked to obesity, physical inactivity, and poor diet. Over time, high blood sugar levels can damage various organs, including the kidneys, leading to or exacerbating CKD.

The relationship between CKD and Diabetes Type 2 is bidirectional. Diabetes can lead to CKD, and CKD can, in turn, contribute to the development or worsening of diabetes. Managing both conditions requires a holistic approach, focusing on diet, exercise, medication, and regular monitoring of blood sugar and kidney function.

The Importance of Diet in Managing CKD and Diabetes

Diet plays a crucial role in managing both Chronic Kidney Disease (CKD) Stage 3 and Diabetes Type 2. Proper nutrition can help slow the progression of CKD, control blood sugar levels, and reduce the risk of complications associated with both conditions.

For individuals with CKD Stage 3, a kidney-friendly diet is essential. This involves limiting certain nutrients that the kidneys may have trouble filtering, such as sodium, potassium, and phosphorus. A diet low in these minerals can help prevent further kidney damage and reduce the risk of other health issues, such as high blood pressure and heart disease.

For those with Diabetes Type 2, a diet that helps control blood sugar levels is vital. This typically includes foods that are low in simple sugars and refined carbohydrates, and high in fiber, lean proteins, and healthy fats. Managing carbohydrate intake and choosing foods with a low glycemic index can help prevent spikes in blood sugar and improve overall glucose control.

Combining the dietary needs of both conditions can be challenging, but it's possible with careful planning and knowledge. This cookbook aims to provide you with recipes that cater to the nutritional requirements of both CKD Stage 3 and Diabetes Type 2, allowing you to enjoy delicious meals while managing your health effectively.

How to Use This Cookbook

This cookbook is designed to be a practical and user-friendly resource for individuals managing both CKD Stage 3 and Diabetes Type 2. Here are some tips on how to get the most out of it:

1. Familiarize Yourself with the Recipes: Take some time to browse through the recipes and note the ones that appeal to you. Each recipe is crafted to be kidney-friendly and diabetes-friendly, providing a balanced combination of nutrients.

2. Plan Your Meals: Use the recipes to plan your meals for the week. This can help you ensure that you have a variety of dishes and that you're meeting your nutritional needs. Consider using the 14-Day Meal Plan provided in the cookbook as a starting point.

3. *Make Adjustments as Needed:* While the recipes are designed to be suitable for CKD Stage 3 and Diabetes Type 2, individual dietary needs may vary. Feel free to adjust the recipes based on your personal preferences and nutritional requirements. For example, you can substitute ingredients or adjust portion sizes as needed.

4. *Cook with Fresh Ingredients:* Whenever possible, use fresh, whole ingredients. This can help you avoid added sugars, sodium, and preservatives, which are often found in processed foods.

5. *Track Your Nutrient Intake:* Pay attention to your intake of key nutrients, such as sodium, potassium, phosphorus, and carbohydrates. This can help you manage your CKD and diabetes more effectively.

6. *Enjoy the Process:* Cooking should be an enjoyable experience. Experiment with different recipes, flavors, and cooking techniques to find what works best for you.

By using this cookbook as a guide, you can create delicious and nutritious meals that support your health and well-being.

Tips for Grocery Shopping and Meal Preparation

Managing CKD Stage 3 and Diabetes Type 2 requires thoughtful grocery shopping and meal preparation. Here are some tips to make the process easier and more efficient:

1. Make a List: Before heading to the grocery store, make a list of the ingredients you need for the recipes you plan to prepare. This can help you stay organized and avoid impulse purchases that may not be suitable for your dietary needs.

2. Read Labels: Pay attention to food labels, especially when buying packaged or processed items. Look for products low in sodium, added sugars, and unhealthy fats. Check for serving sizes and carbohydrate content to help manage your blood sugar levels.

3. Choose Fresh and Whole Foods: Focus on purchasing fresh fruits, vegetables, lean proteins, and whole grains. These foods are generally lower in sodium and higher in nutrients compared to processed foods.

4. *Look for Low-Sodium Options:* If you need to buy canned or packaged foods, look for low-sodium or no-salt-added versions to help manage your sodium intake.

5. *Plan Ahead:* Meal planning can save you time and reduce stress. Prepare and cook meals in advance when you have more time, and store them in the refrigerator or freezer for later use.

6. *Cook in Bulk:* Consider cooking larger quantities of certain dishes or ingredients, such as brown rice or grilled chicken, that can be used in multiple meals throughout the week.

7. *Use Herbs and Spices:* To add flavor without adding sodium, use a variety of herbs and spices in your cooking. Fresh herbs like cilantro, basil, and parsley can enhance the taste of your dishes without compromising your kidney health.

8. *Stay Hydrated:* Drink plenty of water throughout the day to help support kidney function and overall health. Limit sugary drinks and beverages high in phosphorus, such as certain sodas.

By following these tips, you can make grocery shopping and meal preparation more manageable and ensure that your meals are aligned with your dietary needs for managing CKD Stage 3 and Diabetes Type 2.

Key Nutritional Considerations for CKD and Diabetes

When managing CKD Stage 3 and Diabetes Type 2, it's important to understand the key nutritional considerations that can help you maintain your health. Here are some essential points to keep in mind:

1. Carbohydrates: Monitor your carbohydrate intake to manage blood sugar levels. Choose complex carbohydrates like whole grains, fruits, and vegetables, which provide fiber and are absorbed more slowly, helping to prevent spikes in blood sugar.

2. Protein: Moderate your protein intake to reduce the workload on your kidneys. Opt for high-quality protein sources such as lean meats, fish, poultry, and plant-based proteins like beans and lentils.

3. Sodium: Limit sodium intake to help control blood pressure and reduce the risk of kidney damage. Avoid processed and packaged foods, which are often high in sodium, and use herbs and spices to flavor your meals instead of salt.

4. Potassium: Depending on your kidney function, you may need to monitor your potassium intake. Some fruits and vegetables, like bananas and potatoes, are high in potassium and may need to be limited.

5. Phosphorus: High phosphorus levels can cause bone and heart problems in people with CKD. Limit foods high in phosphorus, such as dairy products, nuts, and seeds, and opt for lower-phosphorus alternatives.

6. Fats: Choose healthy fats like olive oil, avocados, and nuts, which can help improve heart health. Avoid trans fats and limit saturated fats, which can contribute to heart disease.

7. Fiber: Increase your fiber intake to help manage blood sugar levels and improve digestive health. Fruits, vegetables, whole grains, and legumes are good sources of fiber.

8. Fluids: Your fluid needs may vary depending on your kidney function. It's important to stay hydrated, but you may need to limit your fluid intake if your kidneys are not able to remove excess fluid effectively.

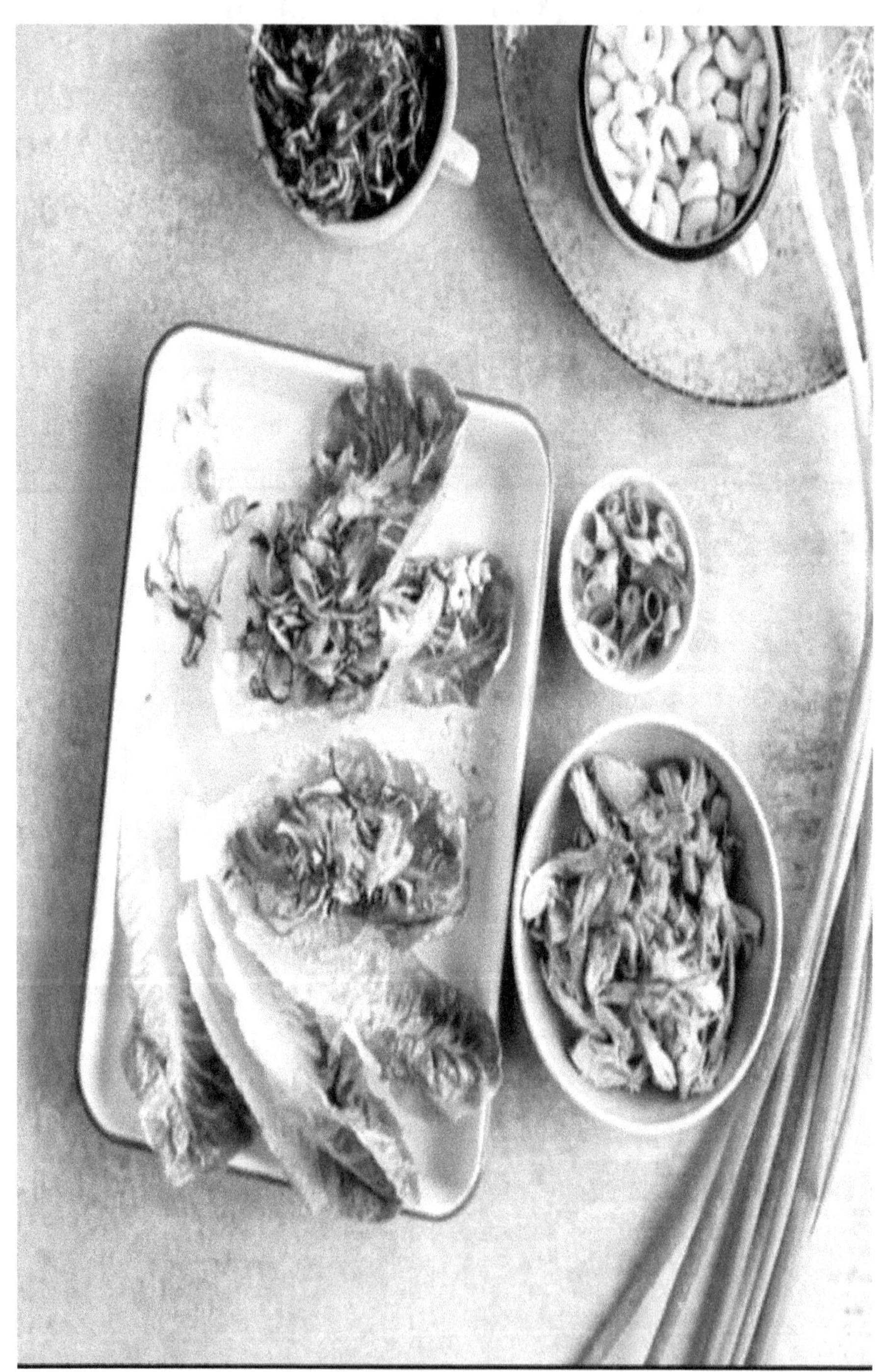

1. Almond and Flaxseed Porridge

- Prep time: 5 minutes

- Cook time: 10 minutes

- Serving size: 1 bowl

Ingredients:

- 1/3 cup rolled oats

- 1 cup unsweetened almond milk

- 1 tablespoon ground flaxseed

- 1/2 teaspoon cinnamon

- 1/4 teaspoon vanilla extract

- 1 tablespoon chopped almonds

- 1 tablespoon sugar-free maple syrup (optional)

Nutritional Facts:

- Calories: 235 kcal

- Carbohydrates: 27g

- Protein: 7g

- Fat: 12g

- Fiber: 6g

- Sodium: 95mg

Preparation Directions:

1. In a small pot, combine the rolled oats and almond milk. Bring to a simmer over medium heat.

2. Stir in the ground flaxseed, cinnamon, and vanilla extract. Cook for about 5-7 minutes, or until the porridge reaches your desired consistency.

3. Pour the porridge into a bowl and top with chopped almonds and a drizzle of sugar-free maple syrup, if desired.

Health Benefit:

This Almond and Flaxseed Porridge is a nutritious breakfast option for individuals with CKD Stage 3 and Diabetes Type 2. The low glycemic index of rolled oats helps in managing blood sugar levels, while the flaxseed provides omega-3 fatty acids that support heart health. Almonds add a healthy dose of protein and fiber, making this porridge a filling and kidney-friendly meal.

2. Spinach and Feta Breakfast Scramble

- *Prep time: 5 minutes*
- *Cook time: 10 minutes*
- *Serving size: 1 serving*

Ingredients:

- 2 large egg whites
- 1 whole egg
- 1/2 cup fresh spinach, chopped
- 1/4 cup crumbled feta cheese
- 1/4 teaspoon black pepper
- 1/2 teaspoon olive oil

Nutritional Facts:

- Calories: 160 kcal
- Carbohydrates: 2g
- Protein: 15g
- Fat: 10g
- Fiber: 0.5g
- Sodium: 320mg

Preparation Directions:

In a medium bowl, whisk together the egg whites, whole egg, and black pepper.

Heat the olive oil in a non-stick skillet over medium heat.

Add the chopped spinach to the skillet and sauté for 1-2 minutes, or until slightly wilted.

Pour the egg mixture into the skillet and cook, stirring gently, until the eggs are set and cooked through.

Sprinkle the crumbled feta cheese over the top of the scrambled eggs and serve.

Health Benefit:

The Spinach and Feta Breakfast Scramble is an excellent source of protein and low in carbohydrates, making it ideal for managing blood sugar levels in Diabetes Type 2 patients. Spinach provides vitamins and minerals, while the feta cheese adds calcium and flavor without adding too much sodium, making it suitable for those with CKD Stage 3.

3. Greek Yogurt with Mixed Berries and Nuts

- *Prep time: 5 minutes*
- *Serving size: 1 bowl*

Ingredients:

- 3/4 cup non-fat Greek yogurt
- 1/2 cup mixed berries (blueberries, raspberries, strawberries)
- 1 tablespoon chopped walnuts
- 1 teaspoon honey (optional)

Nutritional Facts:

- Calories: 180 kcal
- Carbohydrates: 20g
- Protein: 18g
- Fat: 5g
- Fiber: 3g
- Sodium: 60mg

Preparation Directions:

1. In a serving bowl, place the non-fat Greek yogurt.
2. Top the yogurt with the mixed berries.
3. Sprinkle the chopped walnuts over the berries.
4. Drizzle with honey if desired, and serve.

Health Benefit:

This Greek Yogurt with Mixed Berries and Nuts is a refreshing and protein-rich breakfast option. The Greek yogurt provides a good source of protein and probiotics, which are beneficial for gut health. The berries offer antioxidants and fiber, aiding in blood sugar control, while the walnuts provide healthy fats that are good for heart health. This meal is low in sodium, making it suitable for CKD Stage 3 patients.

4. Cauliflower Hash Browns

- Prep time: 10 minutes

- Cook time: 15 minutes

- Serving size: 2 hash browns

Ingredients:

- 2 cups cauliflower rice

- 1 large egg

- 1/4 cup shredded cheddar cheese (low sodium)

- 1/4 teaspoon garlic powder

- 1/4 teaspoon black pepper

- 1 tablespoon olive oil

Nutritional Facts:

- Calories: 190 kcal

- Carbohydrates: 8g

- Protein: 11g

- Fat: 14g

- Fiber: 3g

- Sodium: 180mg

Preparation Directions:

1. In a large bowl, mix together the cauliflower rice, egg, shredded cheddar cheese, garlic powder, and black pepper until well combined.

2. Heat the olive oil in a non-stick skillet over medium heat.

3. Form the cauliflower mixture into small patties and place them in the skillet.

4. Cook for 5-7 minutes on each side, or until they are golden brown and crispy.

5. Remove from the skillet and serve.

Health Benefit:

Cauliflower Hash Browns are a low-carb and kidney-friendly alternative to traditional hash browns. Cauliflower is a low-potassium vegetable, making it suitable for CKD Stage 3 patients. The addition of low-sodium cheddar cheese adds flavor without significantly increasing the sodium content. This recipe is also a good source of protein and healthy fats, which are important for managing Diabetes Type 2.

5. Egg White and Avocado Wrap

- Prep time: 5 minutes

- Cook time: 5 minutes

- Serving size: 1 wrap

Ingredients:

- 3 egg whites

- 1 whole wheat wrap (low sodium)

- 1/4 avocado, sliced

- 1/4 cup baby spinach

- 1 tablespoon salsa (low sodium)

- 1/4 teaspoon black pepper

Nutritional Facts:

- Calories: 220 kcal

- Carbohydrates: 20g

- Protein: 15g

- Fat: 9g

- Fiber: 5g

- Sodium: 240mg

Preparation Directions:

1. In a bowl, whisk the egg whites and black pepper together.

2. Heat a non-stick skillet over medium heat and pour in the egg whites, cooking them until they are set and fully cooked.

3. Warm the whole wheat wrap in the microwave for 10-15 seconds.

4. Place the cooked egg whites on the wrap, and top with sliced avocado, baby spinach, and salsa.

5. Roll up the wrap and serve.

Health Benefit:

The Egg White and Avocado Wrap is a heart-healthy and diabetes-friendly breakfast option. Egg whites are a low-calorie source of protein, which is essential for muscle maintenance and repair. Avocado provides healthy monounsaturated fats that can help improve cholesterol levels. The whole wheat wrap adds fiber, which aids in digestion and blood sugar control, making it a great choice for individuals with CKD Stage 3 and Diabetes Type 2.

6. Low-Glycemic Muesli with Almonds

- *Prep time: 5 minutes*

- *Cook time: 0 minutes*

- *Serving size: 1 bowl*

Ingredients:

- 1/2 cup rolled oats

- 1/4 cup unsweetened almond milk

- 1 tablespoon chia seeds

- 1/4 teaspoon cinnamon

- 1/4 cup sliced almonds

- 1/4 cup diced green apple

- 1 tablespoon sugar-free dried cranberries

Nutritional Facts:

- Calories: 280 kcal

- Carbohydrates: 32g

- Protein: 10g

- Fat: 14g

- Fiber: 8g

- Sodium: 40mg

Preparation Directions:

1. In a bowl, combine the rolled oats, chia seeds, and cinnamon.

2. Add the unsweetened almond milk and mix well.

3. Let the mixture sit for a few minutes to allow the oats and chia seeds to absorb the liquid.

4. Top the muesli with sliced almonds, diced green apple, and sugar-free dried cranberries.

Health Benefit:

Low-Glycemic Muesli with Almonds is a great breakfast choice for those managing CKD Stage 3 and Diabetes Type 2. The low-glycemic index of rolled oats helps maintain stable blood sugar levels, while the chia seeds provide omega-3 fatty acids and fiber for heart health and digestion. Almonds add a crunchy texture and are a good source of healthy fats, protein, and vitamin E.

7. Broccoli and Cheese Mini Quiches

- Prep time: 10 minutes

- Cook time: 20 minutes

- Serving size: 2 mini quiches

Ingredients:

- 1/2 cup chopped broccoli

- 2 large eggs

- 1/4 cup low-fat milk

- 1/4 cup shredded low-sodium cheddar cheese

- 1/4 teaspoon garlic powder

- 1/4 teaspoon black pepper

- Non-stick cooking spray

Nutritional Facts:

- Calories: 160 kcal

- Carbohydrates: 5g

- Protein: 14g

- Fat: 9g

- Fiber: 1g

- Sodium: 180mg

Preparation Directions:

1. Preheat the oven to 375°F (190°C) and lightly spray a muffin tin with non-stick cooking spray.

2. In a bowl, whisk together the eggs, low-fat milk, garlic powder, and black pepper.

3. Divide the chopped broccoli and shredded cheddar cheese evenly among the muffin cups.

4. Pour the egg mixture over the broccoli and cheese, filling each cup about 3/4 full.

5. Bake in the preheated oven for 20 minutes, or until the mini quiches are set and lightly golden on top.

6. Let them cool for a few minutes before removing them from the muffin tin.

Health Benefit:

Broccoli and Cheese Mini Quiches are a nutritious and portion-controlled breakfast option. Broccoli is a low-potassium vegetable, making it suitable for those with CKD Stage 3, and it provides fiber and antioxidants. The eggs and low-sodium cheddar cheese offer high-quality protein and calcium while keeping the sodium content in check, which is essential for managing blood pressure and kidney health.

8. Chia and Pumpkin Seed Pudding

- Prep time: 5 minutes

- Cook time: 0 minutes (plus refrigeration time)

- Serving size: 1 bowl

Ingredients:

- 1/4 cup chia seeds

- 1 cup unsweetened almond milk

- 1 tablespoon pumpkin seeds

- 1/2 teaspoon vanilla extract

- 1/4 teaspoon cinnamon

- 1 tablespoon sugar-free maple syrup (optional)

Nutritional Facts:

- Calories: 220 kcal

- Carbohydrates: 20g

- Protein: 8g

- Fat: 13g

- Fiber: 10g

- Sodium: 90mg

Preparation Directions:

1. In a bowl, combine the chia seeds, unsweetened almond milk, vanilla extract, and cinnamon.
2. Mix well and let the mixture sit for about 5 minutes.
3. Stir again, then cover and refrigerate for at least 2 hours or overnight until the pudding has thickened.
4. Before serving, stir the pudding and top with pumpkin seeds and a drizzle of sugar-free maple syrup, if desired.

Health Benefit:

Chia and Pumpkin Seed Pudding is a fiber-rich breakfast that can aid in digestion and help maintain stable blood sugar levels, which is beneficial for Diabetes Type 2 management. Chia seeds are also high in omega-3 fatty acids, promoting heart health. Pumpkin seeds provide magnesium and zinc, which are important for overall health and can be included in a kidney-friendly diet for those with CKD Stage 3.

9. Turkey Sausage and Veggie Skillet

- Prep time: 10 minutes

- Cook time: 15 minutes

- Serving size: 1 serving

Ingredients:

- 2 turkey sausage links (low sodium), sliced

- 1/2 cup diced bell peppers

- 1/4 cup diced onions

- 1 cup chopped kale

- 1/4 teaspoon black pepper

- 1/2 tablespoon olive oil

Nutritional Facts:

- Calories: 250 kcal

- Carbohydrates: 10g

- Protein: 20g

- Fat: 15g

- Fiber: 2g

- Sodium: 450mg

Preparation Directions:

1. Heat the olive oil in a skillet over medium heat.

2. Add the sliced turkey sausage and cook for about 5 minutes, or until lightly browned.

3. Add the diced bell peppers and onions to the skillet and sauté for another 5 minutes, or until the vegetables are tender.

4. Stir in the chopped kale and cook for an additional 2-3 minutes, or until the kale is wilted.

5. Season with black pepper and serve.

Health Benefit:

The Turkey Sausage and Veggie Skillet is a protein-rich breakfast that provides a good start to the day for those with CKD Stage 3 and Diabetes Type 2. The use of low-sodium turkey sausage helps manage sodium intake, which is important for kidney health. The colorful vegetables, like bell peppers and kale, add vitamins, minerals, and fiber to the meal, supporting overall health and blood sugar control.

10. Oat Bran Pancakes with Blueberries

- Prep time: 10 minutes

- Cook time: 10 minutes

- Serving size: 2 pancakes

Ingredients:

- 1/2 cup oat bran

- 1/2 cup low-fat milk

- 1 large egg

- 1/4 teaspoon baking powder

- 1/4 teaspoon vanilla extract

- 1/2 cup fresh blueberries

- 1 tablespoon sugar-free maple syrup (optional)

Nutritional Facts:

- Calories: 220 kcal

- Carbohydrates: 34g

- Protein: 12g

- Fat: 5g

- Fiber: 7g

- Sodium: 120mg

Preparation Directions:

1. In a bowl, mix together the oat bran, low-fat milk, egg, baking powder, and vanilla extract until well combined.
2. Heat a non-stick skillet over medium heat and lightly coat with cooking spray.
3. Pour 1/4 cup of batter onto the skillet for each pancake.
4. Sprinkle a few blueberries onto each pancake before flipping.
5. Cook for 2-3 minutes on each side, or until golden brown.
6. Serve the pancakes with a drizzle of sugar-free maple syrup, if desired.

Health Benefit:

Oat Bran Pancakes with Blueberries are a heart-healthy and diabetes-friendly breakfast option. Oat bran is high in soluble fiber, which can help lower cholesterol levels and improve blood sugar control. The addition of blueberries provides antioxidants and a natural sweetness, making these pancakes a delicious and nutritious choice for those with CKD Stage 3 and Diabetes Type 2.

---

11. White Bean and Kale Soup

- *Prep time: 10 minutes*

- *Cook time: 25 minutes*

- *Serving size: 1 bowl*

Ingredients:

- 1 tablespoon olive oil

- 1/2 cup diced onions

- 2 cloves garlic, minced

- 4 cups low-sodium vegetable broth

- 1 can (15 oz) white beans, rinsed and drained

- 2 cups chopped kale

- 1/2 teaspoon dried thyme

- 1/4 teaspoon black pepper

- 1 tablespoon lemon juice

Nutritional Facts:

- Calories: 180 kcal

- Carbohydrates: 25g

- Protein: 10g

- Fat: 4g

- Fiber: 6g

- Sodium: 300mg

Preparation Directions:

1. Heat the olive oil in a large pot over medium heat.

2. Add the diced onions and minced garlic, sautéing until the onions are translucent.

3. Pour in the low-sodium vegetable broth and bring to a simmer.

4. Add the white beans, chopped kale, dried thyme, and black pepper.

5. Simmer for about 20 minutes, or until the kale is tender.

6. Stir in the lemon juice and adjust seasoning if necessary.

7. Serve the soup hot.

Health Benefit:

White Bean and Kale Soup is a nutrient-dense and kidney-friendly meal. The low sodium content helps manage blood pressure, while the white beans provide a good source of plant-based protein and fiber, aiding in blood sugar control. Kale is rich in antioxidants and vitamins, supporting overall health. This soup is an excellent choice for those with CKD Stage 3 and Diabetes Type 2.

12. Roasted Red Pepper and Lentil Soup

- Prep time: 10 minutes

- Cook time: 30 minutes

- Serving size: 1 bowl

Ingredients:

- 1 tablespoon olive oil

- 1/2 cup diced onions

- 2 cloves garlic, minced

- 1 jar (12 oz) roasted red peppers, drained and chopped

- 1 cup red lentils, rinsed

- 4 cups low-sodium vegetable broth

- 1/2 teaspoon smoked paprika

- 1/4 teaspoon black pepper

- 1 tablespoon chopped fresh parsley (for garnish)

Nutritional Facts:

- Calories: 210 kcal

- Carbohydrates: 32g

- Protein: 13g

- Fat: 4g

- Fiber: 8g

- Sodium: 320mg

Preparation Directions:

1. Heat the olive oil in a large pot over medium heat.

2. Add the diced onions and minced garlic, sautéing until the onions are translucent.

3. Stir in the chopped roasted red peppers and red lentils.

4. Pour in the low-sodium vegetable broth and bring to a boil.

5. Reduce the heat to low, cover, and simmer for about 25 minutes, or until the lentils are tender.

6. Use an immersion blender to puree the soup until smooth (or blend in batches using a regular blender).

7. Season with smoked paprika and black pepper.

8. Garnish with chopped fresh parsley before serving.

Health Benefit:

Roasted Red Pepper and Lentil Soup is a heartwarming and nutritious meal that's perfect for managing CKD Stage 3 and Diabetes Type 2. The red lentils are an excellent source of protein and fiber, which help stabilize blood sugar levels. The roasted red peppers add a rich flavor and are packed with vitamins A and C. This soup is low in sodium and fat, making it a healthy choice for those with kidney and blood sugar concerns.

13. Arugula and Walnut Salad with Grilled Chicken

- Prep time: 15 minutes

- Cook time: 10 minutes

- Serving size: 1 salad

Ingredients:

- 2 cups arugula

- 4 oz grilled chicken breast, sliced

- 1/4 cup chopped walnuts

- 1/4 cup cherry tomatoes, halved

- 1 tablespoon balsamic vinegar

- 1/2 tablespoon olive oil

- 1/4 teaspoon black pepper

- 1 tablespoon crumbled feta cheese (optional)

Nutritional Facts:

- Calories: 350

- Carbohydrates: 6g

- Protein: 28g

- Fat: 24g

- Fiber: 3g

- Sodium: 200mg

Preparation Directions:

1. Place the arugula in a large salad bowl.

2. Top the arugula with sliced grilled chicken, chopped walnuts, and cherry tomatoes.

3. In a small bowl, whisk together the balsamic vinegar, olive oil, and black pepper to make the dressing.

4. Drizzle the dressing over the salad and toss gently to combine.

5. Sprinkle crumbled feta cheese on top, if desired.

6. Serve the salad immediately.

Health Benefit:

The Arugula and Walnut Salad with Grilled Chicken is a light and protein-rich meal that's ideal for those with CKD Stage 3 and Diabetes Type 2. The lean grilled chicken provides a healthy source of protein, while the arugula and cherry tomatoes offer antioxidants and vitamins. Walnuts add omega-3 fatty acids, which are beneficial for heart health. The salad is dressed with a simple balsamic vinaigrette, keeping the sodium content low.

14. Spinach and Strawberry Salad with Balsamic Vinaigrette

- Prep time: 10 minutes

- Cook time: 0 minutes

- Serving size: 1 salad

Ingredients:

- 2 cups baby spinach

- 1/2 cup sliced strawberries

- 1/4 cup sliced almonds

- 1 tablespoon balsamic vinegar

- 1/2 tablespoon olive oil

- 1/4 teaspoon black pepper

- 1 tablespoon crumbled goat cheese (optional)

Nutritional Facts:

- Calories: 180 kcal

- Carbohydrates: 12g

- Protein: 6g

- Fat: 12g

- Fiber: 4g

- Sodium: 85mg

Preparation Directions:

1. Place the baby spinach in a large salad bowl.

2. Top the spinach with sliced strawberries and sliced almonds.

3. In a small bowl, whisk together the balsamic vinegar, olive oil, and black pepper to make the dressing.

4. Drizzle the dressing over the salad and toss gently to combine.

5. Sprinkle crumbled goat cheese on top, if desired.

6. Serve the salad immediately.

Health Benefit:

The Spinach and Strawberry Salad with Balsamic Vinaigrette is a refreshing and nutrient-packed meal suitable for CKD Stage 3 and Diabetes Type 2 patients. The baby spinach provides a good source of iron and vitamins, while the strawberries add sweetness and antioxidants. Almonds contribute healthy fats and a crunchy texture. The salad is dressed with a heart-healthy balsamic vinaigrette, and the addition of goat cheese adds a creamy texture and calcium.

15. Zucchini Noodle Salad with Lemon Herb Dressing

- Prep time: 15 minutes

- Cook time: 0 minutes

- Serving size: 1 salad

Ingredients:

- 2 cups spiralized zucchini noodles

- 1/4 cup cherry tomatoes, halved

- 1/4 cup cucumber, sliced

- 1 tablespoon chopped fresh basil

- 1 tablespoon chopped fresh parsley

- 1 tablespoon lemon juice

- 1/2 tablespoon olive oil

- 1/4 teaspoon black pepper

- 1 tablespoon crumbled feta cheese (optional)

Nutritional Facts:

- Calories: 120 kcal

- Carbohydrates: 8g

- Protein: 3g

- Fat: 9g

- Fiber: 2g

- Sodium: 115mg

Preparation Directions:

1. Place the spiralized zucchini noodles in a large salad bowl.

2. Add the cherry tomatoes, cucumber slices, chopped basil, and chopped parsley to the bowl.

3. In a small bowl, whisk together the lemon juice, olive oil, and black pepper to make the dressing.

4. Drizzle the dressing over the salad and toss gently to combine.

5. Sprinkle crumbled feta cheese on top, if desired.

6. Serve the salad immediately.

Health Benefit:

The Zucchini Noodle Salad with Lemon Herb Dressing is a light and hydrating meal, perfect for those managing CKD Stage 3 and Diabetes Type 2. Zucchini noodles are a low-carb alternative to traditional pasta, making them ideal for blood sugar control. The fresh herbs and lemon dressing add a burst of flavor and antioxidants, while the feta cheese provides a source of calcium. This salad is low in sodium and calories, supporting overall kidney and heart health.

16. Spicy Pumpkin Soup

- Prep time: 10 minutes

- Cook time: 25 minutes

- Serving size: 1 bowl

Ingredients:

- 1 tablespoon olive oil

- 1/2 cup diced onions

- 2 cloves garlic, minced

- 2 cups pumpkin puree (fresh or canned, unsweetened)

- 3 cups low-sodium vegetable broth

- 1/2 teaspoon ground cumin

- 1/4 teaspoon cayenne pepper (adjust to taste)

- 1/4 teaspoon black pepper

- 1 tablespoon pumpkin seeds (for garnish)

- 1 tablespoon plain Greek yogurt (for garnish, optional)

Nutritional Facts:

- Calories: 150 kcal

- Carbohydrates: 20g

- Protein: 4g

- Fat: 7g

- Fiber: 5g

- Sodium: 200mg

Preparation Directions:

1. Heat the olive oil in a large pot over medium heat.

2. Add the diced onions and minced garlic, sautéing until the onions are translucent.

3. Stir in the pumpkin puree, low-sodium vegetable broth, ground cumin, cayenne pepper, and black pepper.

4. Bring the mixture to a boil, then reduce the heat and simmer for about 20 minutes, allowing the flavors to meld.

5. Use an immersion blender to puree the soup until smooth (or blend in batches using a regular blender).

6. Serve the soup hot, garnished with pumpkin seeds and a dollop of plain Greek yogurt, if desired.

Health Benefit:

Spicy Pumpkin Soup is a warming and nutritious option for individuals with CKD Stage 3 and Diabetes Type 2. Pumpkin is low in potassium and high in fiber, making it kidney-friendly and beneficial for blood sugar control. The addition of cumin and cayenne pepper adds a spicy kick and can help boost metabolism. The soup is low in sodium and calories, supporting overall health and weight management.

17. Asian Chicken Salad with Ginger Sesame Dressing

- Prep time: 15 minutes

- Cook time: 10 minutes

- Serving size: 1 salad

Ingredients:

- 2 cups mixed greens (lettuce, spinach, cabbage)

- 4 oz grilled chicken breast, sliced

- 1/4 cup shredded carrots

- 1/4 cup sliced cucumber

- 1 tablespoon chopped green onions

- 1 tablespoon sesame seeds

Dressing:

- 1 tablespoon soy sauce (low sodium)

- 1 tablespoon rice vinegar

- 1/2 tablespoon sesame oil

- 1/2 teaspoon grated ginger

- 1/4 teaspoon black pepper

Nutritional Facts:

- Calories: 280 kcal

- Carbohydrates: 10g

- Protein: 30g

- Fat: 14g

- Fiber: 3g

- Sodium: 350mg

Preparation Directions:

1. In a large salad bowl, combine the mixed greens, shredded carrots, sliced cucumber, and chopped green onions.

2. Top the salad with sliced grilled chicken and sprinkle with sesame seeds.

3. In a small bowl, whisk together the soy sauce, rice vinegar, sesame oil, grated ginger, and black pepper to make the dressing.

4. Drizzle the dressing over the salad and toss gently to combine.

5. Serve the salad immediately.

Health Benefit:

The Asian Chicken Salad with Ginger Sesame Dressing is a flavorful and balanced meal that's suitable for those with CKD Stage 3 and Diabetes Type 2. The lean grilled chicken provides a good source of protein, while the mixed greens and vegetables offer vitamins, minerals, and fiber. The ginger sesame dressing adds a zesty flavor and has anti-inflammatory properties. This salad is low in sodium and high in nutrients, making it a healthy choice for kidney and blood sugar management.

18. Watermelon and Feta Salad

- Prep time: 10 minutes

- Cook time: 0 minutes

- Serving size: 1 salad

Ingredients:

- 2 cups cubed watermelon

- 1/4 cup crumbled feta cheese

- 1/4 cup sliced red onion

- 1 tablespoon chopped fresh mint

- 1 tablespoon balsamic glaze

- 1/2 tablespoon olive oil

- 1/4 teaspoon black pepper

Nutritional Facts:

- Calories: 180 kcal

- Carbohydrates: 22g

- Protein: 5g

- Fat: 9g

- Fiber: 1g

- Sodium: 250mg

Preparation Directions:

1. In a large salad bowl, combine the cubed watermelon, crumbled feta cheese, sliced red onion, and chopped fresh mint.
2. In a small bowl, whisk together the balsamic glaze, olive oil, and black pepper.
3. Drizzle the dressing over the salad and gently toss to combine.
4. Serve the salad immediately, garnished with additional fresh mint if desired.

Health Benefit:

Watermelon and Feta Salad is a refreshing and hydrating meal, perfect for those with CKD Stage 3 and Diabetes Type 2. Watermelon is low in potassium and provides a natural sweetness, while the feta cheese adds a savory contrast and a source of calcium. The salad is dressed with a balsamic glaze and olive oil, which adds flavor without excess sodium. This salad is light, nutritious, and can help maintain hydration and electrolyte balance.

19. Tomato and Avocado Gazpacho

- Prep time: 15 minutes

- Cook time: 0 minutes (plus chilling time)

- Serving size: 1 bowl

Ingredients:

- 2 cups chopped tomatoes

- 1 ripe avocado, peeled and pitted

- 1/2 cup chopped cucumber

- 1/4 cup chopped red onion

- 1 clove garlic, minced

- 2 tablespoons lime juice

- 1/4 teaspoon cumin

- 1/4 teaspoon black pepper

- 1 cup cold water

- Fresh cilantro (for garnish)

Nutritional Facts:

- Calories: 200 kcal

- Carbohydrates: 18g

- Protein: 4g

- Fat: 14g

- Fiber: 8g

- Sodium: 30mg

Preparation Directions:

1. In a blender, combine the chopped tomatoes, avocado, cucumber, red onion, garlic, lime juice, cumin, black pepper, and cold water.
2. Blend until smooth, adding more water if necessary to reach your desired consistency.
3. Chill the gazpacho in the refrigerator for at least 1 hour before serving.
4. Serve cold, garnished with fresh cilantro.

Health Benefit:

Tomato and Avocado Gazpacho is a cold, refreshing soup that's ideal for CKD Stage 3 and Diabetes Type 2 patients, especially during warmer months. Tomatoes are a good source of lycopene, an antioxidant that supports heart health. Avocado provides healthy fats and fiber, which are beneficial for blood sugar control and heart health. This gazpacho is low in sodium and calories, making it a kidney-friendly and diabetes-friendly option.

20. Cucumber and Radish Salad with Dill Yogurt Dressing

- Prep time: 10 minutes

- Cook time: 0 minutes

- Serving size: 1 salad

Ingredients:

- 1 cup sliced cucumber

- 1/2 cup sliced radishes

- 1/4 cup plain Greek yogurt

- 1 tablespoon chopped fresh dill

- 1 tablespoon lemon juice

- 1/4 teaspoon black pepper

- 1/4 teaspoon garlic powder

Nutritional Facts:

- Calories: 70 kcal

- Carbohydrates: 8g

- Protein: 5g

- Fat: 2g

- Fiber: 2g

- Sodium: 45mg

Preparation Directions:

1. In a large salad bowl, combine the sliced cucumber and radishes.
2. In a small bowl, whisk together the plain Greek yogurt, chopped fresh dill, lemon juice, black pepper, and garlic powder to make the dressing.
3. Pour the dressing over the cucumber and radish slices and toss gently to coat.
4. Serve the salad immediately, garnished with additional fresh dill if desired.

Health Benefit:

Cucumber and Radish Salad with Dill Yogurt Dressing is a light and refreshing meal that's perfect for individuals managing CKD Stage 3 and Diabetes Type 2. Cucumbers and radishes are low in calories and high in water content, promoting hydration and kidney health. The Greek yogurt dressing provides a source of protein and probiotics, which are beneficial for gut health. This salad is low in sodium and carbohydrates, making it a great choice for those looking to manage their blood sugar levels and kidney function.

21. Lemon Herb Grilled Trout

- Prep time: 10 minutes

- Cook time: 8 minutes

- Serving size: 1 fillet

Ingredients:

- 1 trout fillet (about 6 oz)

- 1 tablespoon olive oil

- 1 tablespoon lemon juice

- 1 teaspoon chopped fresh dill

- 1 teaspoon chopped fresh parsley

- 1/4 teaspoon black pepper

- Lemon slices (for garnish)

Nutritional Facts:

- Calories: 230 kcal

- Carbohydrates: 1g

- Protein: 25g

- Fat: 14g

- Fiber: 0g

- Sodium: 60mg

Preparation Directions:

1. Preheat the grill to medium-high heat.
2. In a small bowl, mix together the olive oil, lemon juice, chopped dill, chopped parsley, and black pepper.
3. Brush the mixture onto both sides of the trout fillet.
4. Place the trout on the grill, skin-side down, and grill for about 4 minutes.
5. Carefully flip the trout and grill for an additional 4 minutes, or until the fish flakes easily with a fork.
6. Serve the grilled trout with lemon slices for garnish.

Health Benefit:

Lemon Herb Grilled Trout is a heart-healthy and kidney-friendly main course. Trout is a good source of omega-3 fatty acids, which are beneficial for heart health and inflammation reduction. The use of fresh herbs and lemon adds flavor without the need for excess sodium, making this dish suitable for those with CKD Stage 3 and Diabetes Type 2. The low carbohydrate content also helps in managing blood sugar levels.

22. Turkey and Vegetable Stuffed Peppers

- Prep time: 15 minutes

- Cook time: 30 minutes

- Serving size: 1 stuffed pepper

Ingredients:

- 4 bell peppers, halved and seeded

- 1/2 lb ground turkey

- 1/2 cup diced onions

- 1/2 cup diced zucchini

- 1/2 cup diced mushrooms

- 1 clove garlic, minced

- 1/2 cup low-sodium tomato sauce

- 1/4 teaspoon black pepper

- 1/4 teaspoon dried oregano

- 1/4 cup shredded low-sodium mozzarella cheese

Nutritional Facts:

- Calories: 180 kcal

- Carbohydrates: 12g

- Protein: 15g

- Fat: 8g

- Fiber: 3g

- Sodium: 120mg

Preparation Directions:

1. Preheat the oven to 375°F (190°C).

2. In a skillet over medium heat, cook the ground turkey, onions, zucchini, mushrooms, and garlic until the turkey is browned and the vegetables are tender.

3. Stir in the low-sodium tomato sauce, black pepper, and dried oregano.

4. Place the bell pepper halves in a baking dish, cut-side up.

5. Spoon the turkey and vegetable mixture into the bell pepper halves.

6. Sprinkle shredded mozzarella cheese on top of each stuffed pepper.

7. Bake in the preheated oven for 20-25 minutes, or until the peppers are tender and the cheese is melted.

8. Serve the stuffed peppers hot.

Health Benefit:

Turkey and Vegetable Stuffed Peppers are a nutritious and balanced meal that's ideal for individuals with CKD Stage 3 and Diabetes Type 2. The bell peppers are a good source of vitamins and antioxidants, while the ground turkey provides lean protein.

The addition of vegetables like zucchini and mushrooms increases the fiber content, which is beneficial for digestion and blood sugar control. The low-sodium tomato sauce and mozzarella cheese help keep the sodium content in check, supporting kidney health.

23. Baked Eggplant Parmesan

- Prep time: 15 minutes

- Cook time: 30 minutes

- Serving size: 1 serving

Ingredients:

- 1 medium eggplant, sliced into 1/2-inch rounds

- 1/2 cup whole wheat breadcrumbs

- 1/4 cup grated Parmesan cheese

- 1 teaspoon dried Italian seasoning

- 1/2 cup low-sodium marinara sauce

- 1/2 cup shredded low-sodium mozzarella cheese

- 1 tablespoon olive oil

- 1/4 teaspoon black pepper

Nutritional Facts:

- Calories: 250 kcal

- Carbohydrates: 28g

- Protein: 14g

- Fat: 11g

- Fiber: 8g

- Sodium: 320mg

Preparation Directions:

1. Preheat the oven to 400°F (200°C).

2. In a shallow dish, combine the whole wheat breadcrumbs, grated Parmesan cheese, and dried Italian seasoning.

3. Brush each eggplant slice with olive oil and season with black pepper.

4. Dredge the eggplant slices in the breadcrumb mixture, pressing gently to adhere.

5. Place the breaded eggplant slices on a baking sheet lined with parchment paper.

6. Bake in the preheated oven for 15 minutes, flipping the slices halfway through.

7. Spoon a small amount of low-sodium marinara sauce over each eggplant slice and top with shredded mozzarella cheese.

8. Return to the oven and bake for an additional 10-15 minutes, or until the cheese is melted and bubbly.

9. Serve the Baked Eggplant Parmesan hot, garnished with fresh basil leaves if desired.

Health Benefit:

Baked Eggplant Parmesan is a healthier alternative to the traditional fried version, making it suitable for those with CKD Stage 3 and Diabetes Type 2. Eggplant is a low-calorie vegetable that provides fiber and antioxidants. The whole wheat breadcrumbs offer a healthier source of carbohydrates, and the use of low-sodium marinara sauce and cheeses helps control sodium intake. This dish is a delicious way to enjoy a classic Italian favorite while managing your health.

24. Garlic and Herb Roasted Chicken Thighs

- *Prep time: 10 minutes*
- *Cook time: 35 minutes*
- *Serving size: 2 chicken thighs*

Ingredients:

- 4 chicken thighs, bone-in and skin-on
- 2 tablespoons olive oil
- 3 cloves garlic, minced
- 1 teaspoon dried rosemary
- 1 teaspoon dried thyme
- 1/2 teaspoon black pepper
- 1/2 lemon, sliced (for garnish)

Nutritional Facts:

- Calories: 310 kcal

- Carbohydrates: 2g

- Protein: 22g

- Fat: 24g

- Fiber: 0g

- Sodium: 90mg

Preparation Directions:

1. Preheat the oven to 375°F (190°C).

2. In a small bowl, mix together the olive oil, minced garlic, dried rosemary, dried thyme, and black pepper.

3. Rub the mixture over the chicken thighs, ensuring they are well-coated.

4. Place the chicken thighs on a baking sheet lined with parchment paper.

5. Bake in the preheated oven for 35 minutes, or until the chicken is cooked through and the skin is golden and crispy.

6. Serve the roasted chicken thighs hot, garnished with lemon slices.

Health Benefit:

Garlic and Herb Roasted Chicken Thighs are a flavorful and protein-rich main course that is suitable for those with CKD Stage

3 and Diabetes Type 2. The use of olive oil and herbs provides healthy fats and antioxidants, while the chicken thighs offer a good source of protein, which is important for muscle maintenance and overall health. The low carbohydrate content helps in managing blood sugar levels, making this dish a great option for a satisfying and nutritious meal.

25. Quinoa Stuffed Portobello Mushrooms

- *Prep time: 15 minutes*
- *Cook time: 20 minutes*
- *Serving size: 2 stuffed mushrooms*

Ingredients:

- 4 large Portobello mushroom caps, stems removed

- 1/2 cup cooked quinoa

- 1/4 cup diced red bell pepper

- 1/4 cup diced zucchini

- 2 tablespoons crumbled feta cheese

- 1 tablespoon chopped fresh basil

- 1 tablespoon olive oil

- 1/4 teaspoon black pepper

- 1 tablespoon balsamic vinegar (for drizzling)

Nutritional Facts:

- Calories: 220 kcal

- Carbohydrates: 18g

- Protein: 8g

- Fat: 14g

- Fiber: 4g

- Sodium: 150mg

Preparation Directions:

1. Preheat the oven to 400°F (200°C).

2. In a bowl, combine the cooked quinoa, diced red bell pepper, diced zucchini, crumbled feta cheese, and chopped fresh basil.

3. Brush the Portobello mushroom caps with olive oil and season with black pepper.

4. Spoon the quinoa mixture into the mushroom caps, pressing gently to fill.

5. Place the stuffed mushrooms on a baking sheet lined with parchment paper.

6. Bake in the preheated oven for 20 minutes, or until the mushrooms are tender and the filling is heated through.

7. Drizzle with balsamic vinegar before serving.

Health Benefit:

Quinoa Stuffed Portobello Mushrooms are a vegetarian-friendly and nutrient-dense main course. Quinoa is a complete protein, providing all nine essential amino acids, which is beneficial for those with Diabetes Type 2. The vegetables add fiber and vitamins, while the feta cheese offers calcium. This dish is low in sodium and high in flavor, making it a great choice for managing CKD Stage 3 and maintaining overall health.

26. Shrimp and Cauliflower Grits

- Prep time: 15 minutes

- Cook time: 20 minutes

- Serving size: 1 serving

Ingredients:

- 1 cup riced cauliflower

- 1/2 cup low-sodium chicken broth

- 1/4 cup grated Parmesan cheese

- 1/4 teaspoon garlic powder

- 1/4 teaspoon black pepper

- 6 large shrimp, peeled and deveined

- 1 tablespoon olive oil

- 1 teaspoon paprika

- 1 tablespoon chopped fresh parsley (for garnish)

Nutritional Facts:

- Calories: 280 kcal

- Carbohydrates: 8g

- Protein: 28g

- Fat: 16g

- Fiber: 3g

- Sodium: 390mg

Preparation Directions:

1. In a saucepan, bring the low-sodium chicken broth to a boil.

2. Add the riced cauliflower, reduce the heat to low, and simmer for about 5 minutes, or until tender.

3. Stir in the grated Parmesan cheese, garlic powder, and black pepper. Cook for an additional 2-3 minutes, or until the mixture thickens into a grit-like consistency.

4. In a separate pan, heat the olive oil over medium heat. Season the shrimp with paprika and black pepper.

5. Cook the shrimp for 2-3 minutes on each side, or until they are pink and opaque.

6. Serve the shrimp over the cauliflower grits and garnish with chopped fresh parsley.

Health Benefit:

Shrimp and Cauliflower Grits is a low-carb and kidney-friendly alternative to traditional grits. Cauliflower provides a good source of vitamins and fiber, while the shrimp offers lean protein, which is important for muscle maintenance. The use of low-sodium chicken broth and Parmesan cheese adds flavor without excess sodium, making this dish suitable for those with CKD Stage 3 and Diabetes Type 2. The paprika adds a touch of spice and antioxidants, enhancing the overall nutritional value of the meal.

27. Zucchini Lasagna

- Prep time: 20 minutes

- Cook time: 45 minutes

- Serving size: 1 slice

Ingredients:

- 2 large zucchinis, sliced lengthwise into thin strips

- 1/2 lb lean ground turkey

- 1 cup low-sodium marinara sauce

- 1/2 cup ricotta cheese

- 1/4 cup grated Parmesan cheese

- 1 egg

- 1 teaspoon dried oregano

- 1/2 teaspoon garlic powder

- 1/2 teaspoon black pepper

- 1 cup shredded low-sodium mozzarella cheese

Nutritional Facts:

- Calories: 260 kcal

- Carbohydrates: 12g

- Protein: 25g

- Fat: 14g

- Fiber: 3g

- Sodium: 320mg

Preparation Directions:

1. Preheat the oven to 375°F (190°C).

2. In a skillet over medium heat, cook the ground turkey until browned. Drain any excess fat.

3. Stir in the low-sodium marinara sauce, oregano, garlic powder, and black pepper. Simmer for 5 minutes.

4. In a bowl, mix together the ricotta cheese, grated Parmesan cheese, and egg.

5. In a baking dish, layer the zucchini strips, turkey marinara mixture, and ricotta mixture. Repeat the layers, ending with zucchini strips on top.

6. Sprinkle shredded mozzarella cheese over the top layer of zucchini.

7. Cover with foil and bake in the preheated oven for 30 minutes. Remove the foil and bake for an additional 15 minutes, or until the cheese is melted and bubbly.

8. Let the lasagna cool for a few minutes before slicing and serving.

Health Benefit:

Zucchini Lasagna is a low-carb and nutritious alternative to traditional lasagna, making it an excellent choice for those with CKD Stage 3 and Diabetes Type 2. The zucchini replaces the high-carb lasagna noodles, reducing the overall carbohydrate content, which helps in managing blood sugar levels. Lean ground turkey provides a good source of protein, while the ricotta and mozzarella cheeses offer calcium and protein. The use of low-sodium marinara sauce helps keep the sodium content in check, supporting kidney health.

28. Moroccan Spiced Lamb Chops

- *Prep time: 10 minutes*

- *Cook time: 10 minutes*

- *Serving size: 2 lamb chops*

Ingredients:

- 4 lamb chops

- 1 tablespoon olive oil

- 1 teaspoon ground cumin

- 1 teaspoon paprika

- 1/2 teaspoon ground coriander

- 1/4 teaspoon ground cinnamon

- 1/4 teaspoon black pepper

- 1/4 teaspoon salt (optional)

- Fresh cilantro (for garnish)

Nutritional Facts:

- Calories: 310 kcal

- Carbohydrates: 1g

- Protein: 25g

- Fat: 22g

- Fiber: 0g

- Sodium: 150mg (without added salt)

Preparation Directions:

1. In a small bowl, mix together the olive oil, ground cumin, paprika, ground coriander, ground cinnamon, black pepper, and salt (if using).
2. Rub the spice mixture onto both sides of the lamb chops.
3. Heat a grill or grill pan over medium-high heat.
4. Grill the lamb chops for about 4-5 minutes on each side, or until they reach your desired level of doneness.
5. Serve the lamb chops hot, garnished with fresh cilantro.

Health Benefit:

Moroccan Spiced Lamb Chops are a flavorful and protein-rich main course that can be enjoyed by those with CKD Stage 3 and Diabetes Type 2. Lamb is a good source of protein and iron, which are important for maintaining energy levels and overall health. The blend of spices adds depth of flavor without the need for excess sodium, making this dish a heart-healthy and kidney-friendly option. The use of olive oil provides healthy fats, which are beneficial for heart health.

29. Grilled Tilapia with Mango Salsa

- Prep time: 15 minutes

- Cook time: 10 minutes

- Serving size: 1 fillet with salsa

Ingredients:

- 4 tilapia fillets

- 1 tablespoon olive oil

- 1/4 teaspoon black pepper

- Mango Salsa:

  - 1 cup diced mango

  - 1/4 cup diced red bell pepper

  - 1/4 cup diced red onion

  - 1 tablespoon chopped fresh cilantro

  - 1 tablespoon lime juice

  - 1/4 teaspoon chili powder (optional)

Nutritional Facts:

- Calories: 220 kcal

- Carbohydrates: 12g

- Protein: 25g

- Fat: 8g

- Fiber: 2g

- Sodium: 70mg

Preparation Directions:

1. Preheat the grill to medium-high heat.

2. Brush the tilapia fillets with olive oil and season with black pepper.

3. Grill the tilapia for about 4-5 minutes on each side, or until the fish flakes easily with a fork.

4. In a bowl, combine the diced mango, diced red bell pepper, diced red onion, chopped fresh cilantro, lime juice, and chili powder (if using) to make the mango salsa.

5. Serve the grilled tilapia topped with the mango salsa.

Health Benefit:

Grilled Tilapia with Mango Salsa is a light and refreshing main course that's perfect for those with CKD Stage 3 and Diabetes Type 2. Tilapia is a lean source of protein and low in phosphorus, making it suitable for a kidney-friendly diet. The mango salsa adds a sweet and tangy flavor, along with vitamins A and C. This dish is low in sodium and fat, promoting heart health and helping to manage blood sugar levels.

30. Vegetable and Tofu Stir-Fry with Brown Rice

- *Prep time: 15 minutes*
- *Cook time: 20 minutes*
- *Serving size: 1 serving*

Ingredients:

- 1/2 cup cooked brown rice

- 1/2 block firm tofu, cubed

- 1 tablespoon olive oil

- 1 cup mixed vegetables (broccoli, bell peppers, carrots)

- 2 tablespoons low-sodium soy sauce

- 1 teaspoon grated ginger

- 1 clove garlic, minced

- 1/4 teaspoon black pepper

- 1 tablespoon chopped green onions (for garnish)

- 1 teaspoon sesame seeds (for garnish)

Nutritional Facts:

- Calories: 350 kcal

- Carbohydrates: 38g

- Protein: 18g

- Fat: 16g

- Fiber: 6g

- Sodium: 320mg

Preparation Directions:

1. Heat the olive oil in a large pan or wok over medium-high heat.

2. Add the cubed tofu and cook until golden brown on all sides.

3. Add the mixed vegetables, low-sodium soy sauce, grated ginger, minced garlic, and black pepper to the pan. Stir-fry for about 5-7 minutes, or until the vegetables are tender-crisp.

4. Serve the vegetable and tofu stir-fry over the cooked brown rice.

5. Garnish with chopped green onions and sesame seeds.

Health Benefit:

Vegetable and Tofu Stir-Fry with Brown Rice is a balanced and nutritious meal that's suitable for those with CKD Stage 3 and Diabetes Type 2. The tofu provides a good source of plant-based protein, while the brown rice offers complex carbohydrates for sustained energy. The mixed vegetables contribute vitamins, minerals, and fiber, supporting overall health. This dish is low in sodium and high in flavor, making it a great option for managing kidney health and blood sugar levels.

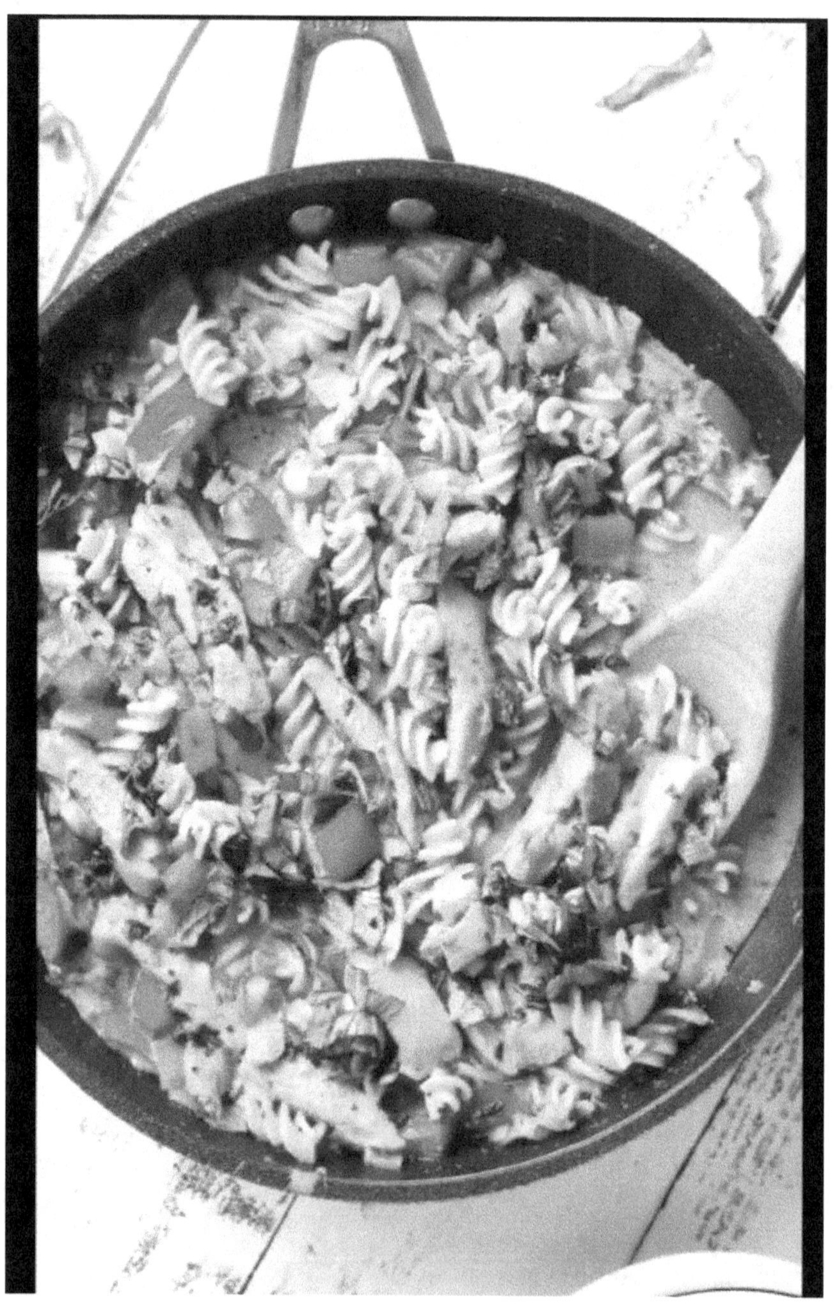

31. Baked Kale Chips with Nutritional Yeast

- Prep time: 5 minutes

- Cook time: 15 minutes

- Serving size: 1 cup

Ingredients:

- 4 cups kale leaves, washed, dried, and torn into bite-sized pieces
- 1 tablespoon olive oil
- 2 tablespoons nutritional yeast
- 1/4 teaspoon garlic powder
- 1/4 teaspoon black pepper

Nutritional Facts:

- Calories: 80 kcal
- Carbohydrates: 8g
- Protcin: 5g
- Fat: 4g
- Fiber: 2g
- Sodium: 50mg

Preparation Directions:

1. Preheat the oven to 350°F (175°C).

2. In a large bowl, toss the kale leaves with olive oil, nutritional yeast, garlic powder, and black pepper until evenly coated.

3. Spread the kale leaves in a single layer on a baking sheet lined with parchment paper.

4. Bake in the preheated oven for 10-15 minutes, or until the kale is crispy and lightly browned.

5. Serve the kale chips immediately or store in an airtight container for later.

Health Benefit:

Baked Kale Chips with Nutritional Yeast are a nutritious and low-calorie snack that's ideal for those with CKD Stage 3 and Diabetes Type 2. Kale is rich in vitamins A, C, and K, as well as antioxidants that support overall health. Nutritional yeast adds a cheesy flavor and provides additional protein and B vitamins. This snack is low in sodium and carbohydrates, making it a great choice for managing blood sugar levels and kidney health.

32. Roasted Brussels Sprouts with Balsamic Glaze

- Prep time: 10 minutes

- Cook time: 25 minutes

- Serving size: 1/2 cup

Ingredients:

- 2 cups Brussels sprouts, halved

- 1 tablespoon olive oil

- 1/4 teaspoon black pepper

- 2 tablespoons balsamic glaze

Nutritional Facts:

- Calories: 90 kcal

- Carbohydrates: 11g

- Protein: 3g

- Fat: 4g

- Fiber: 3g

- Sodium: 25mg

Preparation Directions:

1. Preheat the oven to 400°F (200°C).

2. Toss the Brussels sprouts with olive oil and black pepper until evenly coated.

3. Spread the Brussels sprouts in a single layer on a baking sheet lined with parchment paper.

4. Roast in the preheated oven for 20-25 minutes, or until the Brussels sprouts are tender and caramelized.

5. Drizzle with balsamic glaze before serving.

Health Benefit:

Roasted Brussels Sprouts with Balsamic Glaze are a delicious and healthy side dish that's suitable for those with CKD Stage 3 and Diabetes Type 2. Brussels sprouts are a good source of fiber, vitamins, and antioxidants, which support overall health. The balsamic glaze adds a touch of sweetness without adding too much sugar, making this dish a great option for managing blood sugar levels. The low sodium content also makes it a kidney-friendly choice.

33. Garlic and Thyme Roasted Carrots

- *Prep time: 10 minutes*

- *Cook time: 25 minutes*

- *Serving size: 1/2 cup*

Ingredients:

- 2 cups baby carrots

- 1 tablespoon olive oil

- 2 cloves garlic, minced

- 1 teaspoon dried thyme

- 1/4 teaspoon black pepper

Nutritional Facts:

- Calories: 70 kcal

- Carbohydrates: 9g

- Protein: 1g

- Fat: 3g

- Fiber: 2g

- Sodium: 45mg

Preparation Directions:

1. Preheat the oven to 400°F (200°C).

2. In a bowl, toss the baby carrots with olive oil, minced garlic, dried thyme, and black pepper until evenly coated.

3. Spread the carrots in a single layer on a baking sheet lined with parchment paper.

4. Roast in the preheated oven for 20-25 minutes, or until the carrots are tender and slightly caramelized.

5. Serve the roasted carrots hot as a side dish.

Health Benefit:

Garlic and Thyme Roasted Carrots are a flavorful and nutritious side dish that's perfect for those with CKD Stage 3 and Diabetes Type 2. Carrots are a good source of beta-carotene, fiber, and vitamins, which support eye health and digestion. The addition of garlic and thyme adds flavor without the need for excess sodium, making this dish a great choice for maintaining kidney health. The low carbohydrate content also helps in managing blood sugar levels.

34. Cucumber and Mint Yogurt Dip

- Prep time: 10 minutes

- Serving size: 2 tablespoons

Ingredients:

- 1 cup plain Greek yogurt

- 1/2 cup finely diced cucumber

- 1 tablespoon chopped fresh mint

- 1 clove garlic, minced

- 1 tablespoon lemon juice

- 1/4 teaspoon black pepper

Nutritional Facts:

- Calories: 30 kcal

- Carbohydrates: 3g

- Protein: 4g

- Fat: 0g

- Fiber: 0g

- Sodium: 15mg

Preparation Directions:

1. In a bowl, mix together the plain Greek yogurt, finely diced cucumber, chopped fresh mint, minced garlic, lemon juice, and black pepper.

2. Cover and refrigerate the dip for at least 30 minutes to allow the flavors to meld.

3. Serve the cucumber and mint yogurt dip as a refreshing side or snack with fresh vegetables or whole-grain crackers.

Health Benefit:

Cucumber and Mint Yogurt Dip is a light and healthy snack that's ideal for those with CKD Stage 3 and Diabetes Type 2. The Greek yogurt provides a good source of protein and probiotics, which are beneficial for gut health. Cucumber adds a refreshing crunch and helps with hydration, while mint adds a fresh flavor. This dip is low in sodium and carbohydrates, making it a great choice for managing kidney health and blood sugar levels.

35. Spiced Roasted Almonds

- Prep time: 5 minutes

- Cook time: 10 minutes

- Serving size: 1/4 cup

Ingredients:

- 1 cup raw almonds

- 1 tablespoon olive oil

- 1/2 teaspoon paprika

- 1/4 teaspoon garlic powder

- 1/4 teaspoon black pepper

- 1/4 teaspoon cayenne pepper (optional)

Nutritional Facts:

- Calories: 170 kcal

- Carbohydrates: 6g

- Protein: 6g

- Fat: 15g

- Fiber: 3g

- Sodium: 0mg

Preparation Directions:

1. Preheat the oven to 350°F (175°C).

2. In a bowl, toss the raw almonds with olive oil, paprika, garlic powder, black pepper, and cayenne pepper (if using) until evenly coated.

3. Spread the almonds in a single layer on a baking sheet lined with parchment paper.

4. Roast in the preheated oven for 10 minutes, stirring halfway through, until the almonds are lightly toasted.

5. Let the almonds cool before serving or storing in an airtight container.

Health Benefit:

Spiced Roasted Almonds are a heart-healthy and satisfying snack that's suitable for those with CKD Stage 3 and Diabetes Type 2. Almonds are a good source of healthy fats, protein, and fiber, which can help manage cholesterol levels and keep you feeling full. The spices add flavor without adding sodium, making this snack a great option for maintaining kidney health. The low carbohydrate content also helps in managing blood sugar levels.

36. Grilled Asparagus with Lemon Zest

- Prep time: 5 minutes

- Cook time: 8 minutes

- Serving size: 1/2 cup

Ingredients:

- 2 cups asparagus spears, trimmed

- 1 tablespoon olive oil

- 1/4 teaspoon black pepper

- 1/2 lemon, zested

Nutritional Facts:

- Calories: 60 kcal

- Carbohydrates: 4g

- Protein: 2g

- Fat: 4g

- Fiber: 2g

- Sodium: 0mg

Preparation Directions:

1. Preheat the grill to medium-high heat.

2. Toss the asparagus spears with olive oil and black pepper.

3. Grill the asparagus for about 4 minutes on each side, or until they are tender and slightly charred.

4. Remove the asparagus from the grill and sprinkle with lemon zest.

5. Serve the grilled asparagus as a side dish or snack.

Health Benefit:

Grilled Asparagus with Lemon Zest is a light and nutritious side dish that's perfect for those with CKD Stage 3 and Diabetes Type 2. Asparagus is low in potassium and high in fiber, making it a kidney-friendly vegetable. The addition of lemon zest adds a refreshing flavor and provides vitamin C. This dish is low in sodium and calories, supporting overall health and blood sugar management.

37. Edamame Salad with Cherry Tomatoes

- Prep time: 10 minutes

- Serving size: 1/2 cup

Ingredients:

- 1 cup shelled edamame, cooked and cooled

- 1/2 cup cherry tomatoes, halved

- 1 tablespoon olive oil

- 1 tablespoon lemon juice

- 1/4 teaspoon black pepper

- 1 tablespoon chopped fresh basil

Nutritional Facts:

- Calories: 120 kcal

- Carbohydrates: 8g

- Protein: 8g

- Fat: 7g

- Fiber: 4g

- Sodium: 15mg

Preparation Directions:

1. In a bowl, combine the cooked and cooled shelled edamame and halved cherry tomatoes.
2. In a small bowl, whisk together the olive oil, lemon juice, and black pepper.
3. Pour the dressing over the edamame and cherry tomatoes, tossing gently to coat.
4. Sprinkle the salad with chopped fresh basil before serving.

Health Benefit:

Edamame Salad with Cherry Tomatoes is a protein-rich and colorful snack or side dish that's suitable for those with CKD Stage 3 and Diabetes Type 2. Edamame provides a good source of plant-based protein and fiber, which can help manage blood sugar levels and support kidney health. Cherry tomatoes add a burst of flavor and are a good source of vitamins and antioxidants. The salad is dressed with a simple olive oil and lemon juice dressing, keeping it low in sodium and calories.

38. Avocado and Black Bean Dip

- Prep time: 10 minutes

- Serving size: 2 tablespoons

Ingredients:

- 1 ripe avocado, mashed

- 1/2 cup black beans, rinsed and drained

- 1 tablespoon lime juice

- 1/4 teaspoon garlic powder

- 1/4 teaspoon cumin

- 1/4 teaspoon black pepper

- 1 tablespoon chopped fresh cilantro

Nutritional Facts:

- Calories: 50 kcal

- Carbohydrates: 5g

- Protein: 2g

- Fat: 3g

- Fiber: 2g

- Sodium: 10mg

Preparation Directions:

1. In a bowl, mash the ripe avocado until smooth.

2. Add the black beans, lime juice, garlic powder, cumin, and black pepper to the mashed avocado. Mix well to combine.

3. Stir in the chopped fresh cilantro.

4. Serve the avocado and black bean dip with fresh vegetables or whole-grain crackers as a healthy snack or appetizer.

Health Benefit:

Avocado and Black Bean Dip is a heart-healthy and kidney-friendly snack that's perfect for those with CKD Stage 3 and Diabetes Type 2. Avocado provides healthy fats and fiber, which can help improve cholesterol levels and aid in digestion. Black beans are a good source of plant-based protein and fiber, supporting blood sugar control and kidney health. The dip is low in sodium and high in flavor, making it a great choice for a nutritious and satisfying snack.

39. Green Bean and Almond Salad

- *Prep time: 10 minutes*

- *Cook time: 5 minutes*

- *Serving size: 1/2 cup*

Ingredients:

- 2 cups green beans, trimmed and blanched

- 1/4 cup sliced almonds, toasted

- 1 tablespoon olive oil

- 1 tablespoon lemon juice

- 1/4 teaspoon black pepper

- 1 tablespoon chopped fresh parsley

Nutritional Facts:

- Calories: 80 kcal

- Carbohydrates: 6g

- Protein: 3g

- Fat: 6g

- Fiber: 3g

- Sodium: 10mg

Preparation Directions:

1. Blanch the green beans in boiling water for 2-3 minutes, then plunge them into ice water to stop the cooking process. Drain well.

2. In a bowl, combine the blanched green beans and toasted sliced almonds.

3. In a small bowl, whisk together the olive oil, lemon juice, and black pepper.

4. Pour the dressing over the green bean and almond mixture, tossing gently to coat.

5. Sprinkle the salad with chopped fresh parsley before serving.

Health Benefit:

Green Bean and Almond Salad is a crunchy and nutritious side dish that's suitable for those with CKD Stage 3 and Diabetes Type 2. Green beans are a low-potassium vegetable that provides fiber and vitamins, while almonds add a good source of healthy fats and protein. The salad is dressed with a simple olive oil and lemon juice dressing, keeping it low in sodium and calories. This dish is a great way to add more vegetables and healthy fats to your diet while managing kidney health and blood sugar levels.

40. Celery Sticks with Almond Butter

- *Prep time: 5 minutes*

- *Cook time: 0 minutes*

- *Serving size: 2 celery sticks with 1 tablespoon almond butter*

Ingredients:

- 4 celery sticks, washed and cut into 3-inch pieces

- 2 tablespoons almond butter

Nutritional Facts:

- Calories: 100 kcal

- Carbohydrates: 4g

- Protein: 3g

- Fat: 8g

- Fiber: 2g

- Sodium: 40mg

Preparation Directions:

1. Spread 1/2 tablespoon of almond butter onto each celery stick.

2. Serve the celery sticks with almond butter as a healthy and crunchy snack.

Health Benefit:

Celery Sticks with Almond Butter are a simple and nutritious snack that's ideal for those with CKD Stage 3 and Diabetes Type 2. Celery is a low-calorie and low-potassium vegetable that provides hydration and fiber. Almond butter is a good source of healthy fats and protein, which can help manage blood sugar levels and provide sustained energy. This snack is low in sodium and carbohydrates, making it a great choice for managing kidney health and blood sugar levels.

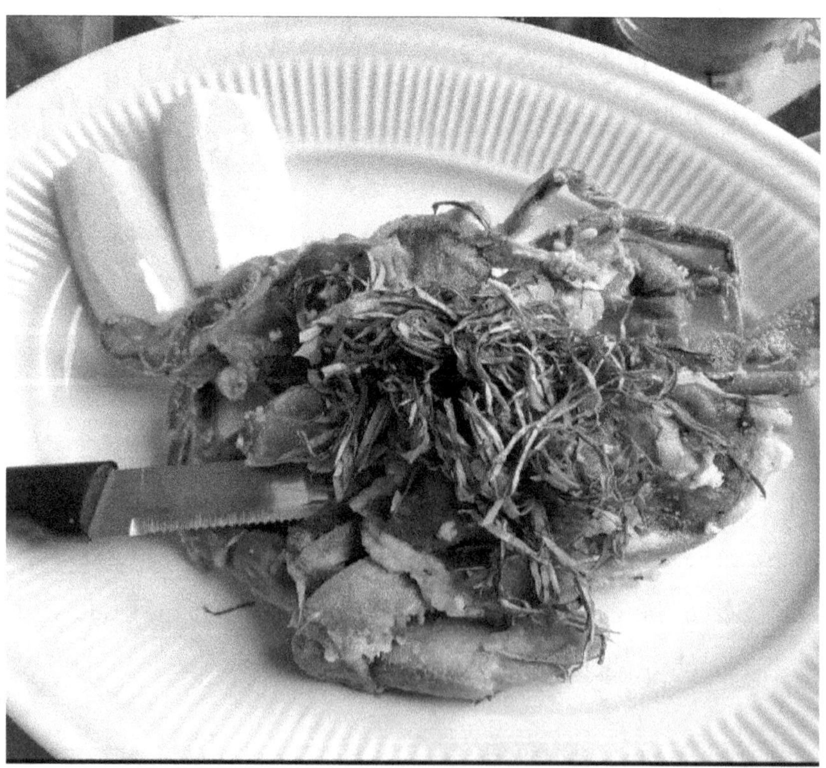

41. Baked Pears with Cinnamon and Walnuts

- *Prep time: 10 minutes*
- *Cook time: 25 minutes*
- *Serving size: 1/2 pear*

Ingredients:

- 2 ripe pears, halved and cored
- 1 teaspoon ground cinnamon
- 1/4 cup chopped walnuts
- 1 tablespoon honey (optional)

Nutritional Facts:

- Calories: 110 kcal
- Carbohydrates: 19g
- Protein: 2g
- Fat: 4g
- Fiber: 4g
- Sodium: 0mg

Preparation Directions:

1. Preheat the oven to 350°F (175°C).

2. Place the pear halves cut-side up in a baking dish.

3. Sprinkle the pears with ground cinnamon and top with chopped walnuts.

4. Drizzle honey over the pears, if using.

5. Bake in the preheated oven for 25 minutes, or until the pears are tender and the walnuts are toasted.

6. Serve the baked pears warm as a guilt-free dessert.

Health Benefit:

Baked Pears with Cinnamon and Walnuts are a delicious and healthy dessert option for those with CKD Stage 3 and Diabetes Type 2. Pears are a good source of fiber and vitamins, while cinnamon adds flavor and may help regulate blood sugar levels. Walnuts provide healthy fats and protein. This dessert is low in sodium and can be made without added sugars, making it a great choice for managing kidney health and blood sugar levels.

42. Raspberry and Almond Flour Muffins

- Prep time: 10 minutes

- Cook time: 20 minutes

- Serving size: 1 muffin

Ingredients:

- 1 1/2 cups almond flour

- 1/2 cup granulated erythritol (or sweetener of choice)

- 2 teaspoons baking powder

- 1/4 teaspoon salt

- 3 large eggs

- 1/3 cup unsweetened almond milk

- 1/4 cup melted coconut oil

- 1 teaspoon vanilla extract

- 1/2 cup fresh raspberries

Nutritional Facts:

- Calories: 160 kcal

- Carbohydrates: 8g (net carbs)

- Protein: 6g

- Fat: 13g

- Fiber: 3g

- Sodium: 150mg

Preparation Directions:

1. Preheat the oven to 350°F (175°C) and line a muffin tin with paper liners.

2. In a large bowl, mix together the almond flour, erythritol, baking powder, and salt.

3. In a separate bowl, whisk together the eggs, almond milk, melted coconut oil, and vanilla extract.

4. Add the wet ingredients to the dry ingredients and stir until just combined.

5. Gently fold in the fresh raspberries.

6. Divide the batter evenly among the muffin cups.

7. Bake in the preheated oven for 18-20 minutes, or until a toothpick inserted into the center of a muffin comes out clean.

8. Allow the muffins to cool in the pan for 5 minutes before transferring them to a wire rack to cool completely.

Health Benefit:

Raspberry and Almond Flour Muffins are a low-carb and gluten-free dessert option that's suitable for those with CKD Stage 3 and Diabetes Type 2. Almond flour provides a good source of healthy fats and protein, while raspberries add natural sweetness and are high in antioxidants. The use of a sugar substitute like erythritol helps keep the carbohydrate content low, making these muffins a great choice for managing blood sugar levels.

43. Dark Chocolate Avocado Truffles

- Prep time: 15 minutes

- Cook time: 0 minutes (plus chilling time)

- Serving size: 1 truffle

Ingredients:

- 1 ripe avocado, mashed

- 1/2 cup dark chocolate, melted

- 1 tablespoon cocoa powder (for coating)

- 1/4 teaspoon vanilla extract

Nutritional Facts:

- Calories: 60 kcal

- Carbohydrates: 4g

- Protein: 1g

- Fat: 5g

- Fiber: 2g

- Sodium: 0mg

Preparation Directions:

1. In a bowl, mix together the mashed avocado, melted dark chocolate, and vanilla extract until smooth.
2. Chill the mixture in the refrigerator for about 30 minutes, or until it is firm enough to handle.
3. Using a spoon or melon baller, scoop out small portions of the mixture and roll them into balls.
4. Roll each truffle in cocoa powder to coat.
5. Place the truffles on a plate or tray and chill in the refrigerator until firm.
6. Serve the dark chocolate avocado truffles as a guilt-free dessert.

Health Benefit:

Dark Chocolate Avocado Truffles are a rich and creamy dessert that's perfect for those with CKD Stage 3 and Diabetes Type 2. Avocado provides healthy fats and fiber, while dark chocolate is a good source of antioxidants. These truffles are low in sodium and can be made with a sugar-free dark chocolate to reduce the carbohydrate content, making them a great choice for managing blood sugar levels and kidney health.

44. Coconut Chia Seed Pudding

- *Prep time: 5 minutes*

- *Cook time: 0 minutes (plus chilling time)*

- *Serving size: 1/2 cup*

Ingredients:

- 1/4 cup chia seeds

- 1 cup unsweetened coconut milk

- 1 tablespoon sugar-free sweetener (optional)

- 1/2 teaspoon vanilla extract

- 1/4 cup fresh berries (for topping)

Nutritional Facts:

- Calories: 140 kcal

- Carbohydrates: 10g

- Protein: 4g

- Fat: 10g

- Fiber: 6g

- Sodium: 15mg

Preparation Directions:

1. In a bowl, mix together the chia seeds, unsweetened coconut milk, sugar-free sweetener (if using), and vanilla extract.

2. Stir well to combine and ensure there are no clumps of chia seeds.

3. Cover the bowl and refrigerate for at least 2 hours or overnight, until the pudding has thickened and the chia seeds have absorbed the liquid.

4. Stir the pudding before serving and top with fresh berries.

Health Benefit:

Coconut Chia Seed Pudding is a nutritious and filling dessert that's suitable for those with CKD Stage 3 and Diabetes Type 2. Chia seeds are high in fiber and omega-3 fatty acids, which can help improve heart health and digestion. The use of unsweetened coconut milk keeps the pudding low in carbohydrates and sugars, making it a great option for managing blood sugar levels. The addition of fresh berries adds natural sweetness and antioxidants, enhancing the overall nutritional value of the dessert.

45. Grilled Pineapple with Cinnamon Honey Drizzle

- *Prep time: 5 minutes*
- *Cook time: 10 minutes*
- *Serving size: 1 slice*

Ingredients:

- 4 pineapple slices, about 1/2 inch thick
- 1 tablespoon honey
- 1/2 teaspoon ground cinnamon
- 1/4 teaspoon vanilla extract

Nutritional Facts:

- Calories: 70 kcal
- Carbohydrates: 18g
- Protein: 1g
- Fat: 0g
- Fiber: 2g
- Sodium: 0mg

Preparation Directions:

1. Preheat the grill to medium-high heat.

2. In a small bowl, mix together the honey, ground cinnamon, and vanilla extract.

3. Grill the pineapple slices for about 5 minutes on each side, or until they are slightly charred and tender.

4. Remove the pineapple slices from the grill and drizzle with the cinnamon honey mixture.

5. Serve the grilled pineapple warm as a guilt-free dessert.

Health Benefit:

Grilled Pineapple with Cinnamon Honey Drizzle is a simple and delicious dessert that's perfect for those with CKD Stage 3 and Diabetes Type 2. Pineapple is a good source of vitamins and antioxidants, while cinnamon adds flavor and may help regulate blood sugar levels. The use of honey provides natural sweetness in moderation. This dessert is low in fat and sodium, making it a great choice for maintaining kidney health and managing blood sugar levels.

46. Blueberry and Lemon Sorbet

- Prep time: 10 minutes

- Cook time: 0 minutes (plus freezing time)

- Serving size: 1/2 cup

Ingredients:

- 2 cups fresh or frozen blueberries

- 1/4 cup fresh lemon juice

- 1/4 cup water

- 1/4 cup sugar-free sweetener (optional)

- Lemon zest (for garnish)

Nutritional Facts:

- Calories: 50 kcal

- Carbohydrates: 12g

- Protein: 1g

- Fat: 0g

- Fiber: 2g

- Sodium: 0mg

Preparation Directions:

1. In a blender, combine the blueberries, lemon juice, water, and sugar-free sweetener (if using). Blend until smooth.

2. Pour the mixture into a shallow dish or ice cream maker and freeze according to the manufacturer's instructions.

3. If using a dish, stir the mixture every 30 minutes to break up any ice crystals, until the sorbet is firm but scoopable.

4. Serve the blueberry and lemon sorbet in bowls, garnished with lemon zest.

Health Benefit:

Blueberry and Lemon Sorbet is a refreshing and antioxidant-rich dessert that's ideal for those with CKD Stage 3 and Diabetes Type 2. Blueberries are low in potassium and high in antioxidants, which can help protect against oxidative stress. Lemon adds a tangy flavor and vitamin C, while the use of a sugar-free sweetener helps keep the carbohydrate content low, making this sorbet a great option for managing blood sugar levels.

47. No-Bake Peanut Butter and Oat Bars

- Prep time: 10 minutes

- Cook time: 0 minutes (plus chilling time)

- Serving size: 1 bar

Ingredients:

- 1 cup rolled oats

- 1/2 cup natural peanut butter

- 1/4 cup sugar-free sweetener (optional)

- 1/4 cup unsweetened almond milk

- 1 teaspoon vanilla extract

- 1/4 teaspoon salt

Nutritional Facts:

- Calories: 120 kcal

- Carbohydrates: 10g

- Protein: 4g

- Fat: 8g

- Fiber: 2g

- Sodium: 75mg

Preparation Directions:

1. In a bowl, mix together the rolled oats, peanut butter, sugar-free sweetener (if using), almond milk, vanilla extract, and salt until well combined.

2. Line a small baking dish or tray with parchment paper.

3. Press the oat mixture firmly into the prepared dish, creating an even layer.

4. Chill in the refrigerator for at least 1 hour, or until the bars are firm.

5. Cut the chilled mixture into bars and serve as a guilt-free dessert or snack.

Health Benefit:

No-Bake Peanut Butter and Oat Bars are a convenient and satisfying dessert that's suitable for those with CKD Stage 3 and Diabetes Type 2. The rolled oats provide a good source of fiber, which can help manage blood sugar levels. Natural peanut butter adds healthy fats and protein, making these bars a filling and nutritious option. The use of a sugar-free sweetener and unsweetened almond milk keeps the bars low in sugar and carbohydrates.

48. Kiwi and Lime Frozen Yogurt

- Prep time: 10 minutes

- Cook time: 0 minutes (plus freezing time)

- Serving size: 1/2 cup

Ingredients:

- 2 cups plain Greek yogurt

- 4 ripe kiwis, peeled and chopped

- 1/4 cup fresh lime juice

- 1/4 cup sugar-free sweetener (optional)

- Lime zest (for garnish)

Nutritional Facts:

- Calories: 90 kcal

- Carbohydrates: 10g

- Protein: 9g

- Fat: 1g

- Fiber: 1g

- Sodium: 30mg

Preparation Directions:

1. In a blender, combine the plain Greek yogurt, chopped kiwis, lime juice, and sugar-free sweetener (if using). Blend until smooth.

2. Pour the mixture into an ice cream maker and freeze according to the manufacturer's instructions.

3. If you don't have an ice cream maker, pour the mixture into a shallow dish and freeze, stirring every 30 minutes to break up any ice crystals, until the frozen yogurt is firm but scoopable.

4. Serve the kiwi and lime frozen yogurt in bowls, garnished with lime zest.

Health Benefit:

Kiwi and Lime Frozen Yogurt is a tangy and vitamin-rich dessert that's perfect for those with CKD Stage 3 and Diabetes Type 2. Greek yogurt provides a good source of protein and probiotics, which can support digestive health. Kiwi is low in potassium and high in vitamin C, making it a kidney-friendly fruit. The use of a sugar-free sweetener and the natural sweetness of the kiwi help keep the dessert low in sugar, making it a great option for managing blood sugar levels.

49. Almond and Orange Zest Biscotti

- *Prep time: 15 minutes*

- *Cook time: 40 minutes*

- *Serving size: 1 biscotti*

Ingredients:

- 1 1/2 cups almond flour

- 1/2 cup granulated erythritol (or sweetener of choice)

- 1 teaspoon baking powder

- 1/4 teaspoon salt

- 2 large eggs

- 1 teaspoon vanilla extract

- 1 tablespoon orange zest

- 1/4 cup sliced almonds

Nutritional Facts:

- Calories: 100 kcal

- Carbohydrates: 4g (net carbs)

- Protein: 4g

- Fat: 8g

- Fiber: 2g

- Sodium: 80mg

Preparation Directions:

1. Preheat the oven to 350°F (175°C) and line a baking sheet with parchment paper.
2. In a large bowl, mix together the almond flour, erythritol, baking powder, and salt.
3. In a separate bowl, whisk together the eggs, vanilla extract, and orange zest.
4. Add the wet ingredients to the dry ingredients and mix until well combined.
5. Stir in the sliced almonds.
6. Form the dough into a log shape on the prepared baking sheet.
7. Bake in the preheated oven for 20 minutes, or until the log is firm to the touch.
8. Remove from the oven and let cool for 10 minutes.
9. Using a serrated knife, slice the log diagonally into biscotti.
10. Return the biscotti to the baking sheet, cut-side down, and bake for an additional 10-15 minutes, or until they are crisp and golden.
11. Let the biscotti cool completely on a wire rack before serving.

Health Benefit:

Almond and Orange Zest Biscotti are a delightful and low-carb dessert option that's suitable for those with CKD Stage 3 and Diabetes Type 2. Almond flour provides a gluten-free and low-glycemic base, while the orange zest adds a refreshing citrus flavor. The use of a sugar substitute like erythritol helps keep the biscotti low in sugar, making them a great choice for managing blood sugar levels. The addition of sliced almonds adds a crunchy texture and healthy fats.

50. Strawberry and Basil Salad with Balsamic Reduction

- Prep time: 10 minutes

- Cook time: 10 minutes (for balsamic reduction)

- Serving size: 1/2 cup

Ingredients:

- 2 cups fresh strawberries, hulled and halved

- 1/4 cup fresh basil leaves, torn

- 1/2 cup balsamic vinegar (for reduction)

- 1 tablespoon sugar-free sweetener (optional)

Nutritional Facts:

- Calories: 50 kcal

- Carbohydrates: 12g

- Protein: 1g

- Fat: 0g

- Fiber: 2g

- Sodium: 5mg

Preparation Directions:

1. To make the balsamic reduction, pour the balsamic vinegar into a small saucepan and add the sugar-free sweetener (if using).

2. Bring the mixture to a boil, then reduce the heat and simmer for about 10 minutes, or until the vinegar has reduced by half and has a syrupy consistency.

3. Allow the balsamic reduction to cool.

4. In a salad bowl, combine the fresh strawberries and torn basil leaves.

5. Drizzle the balsamic reduction over the strawberry and basil salad before serving.

Health Benefit:

Strawberry and Basil Salad with Balsamic Reduction is a light and refreshing dessert that's perfect for those with CKD Stage 3 and

Diabetes Type 2. Strawberries are low in potassium and high in antioxidants, making them a kidney-friendly fruit. Basil adds a fresh and aromatic flavor, while the balsamic reduction provides a sweet and tangy dressing without the need for added sugars. This dessert is low in sodium and calories, making it a great choice for managing blood sugar levels and kidney health.

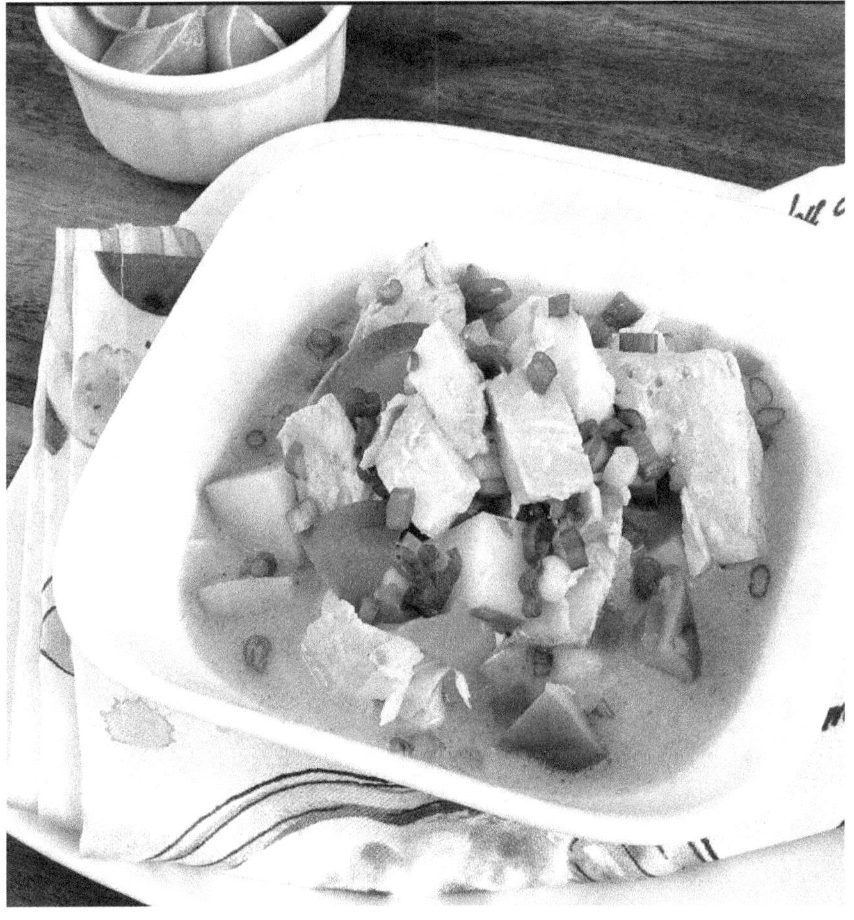

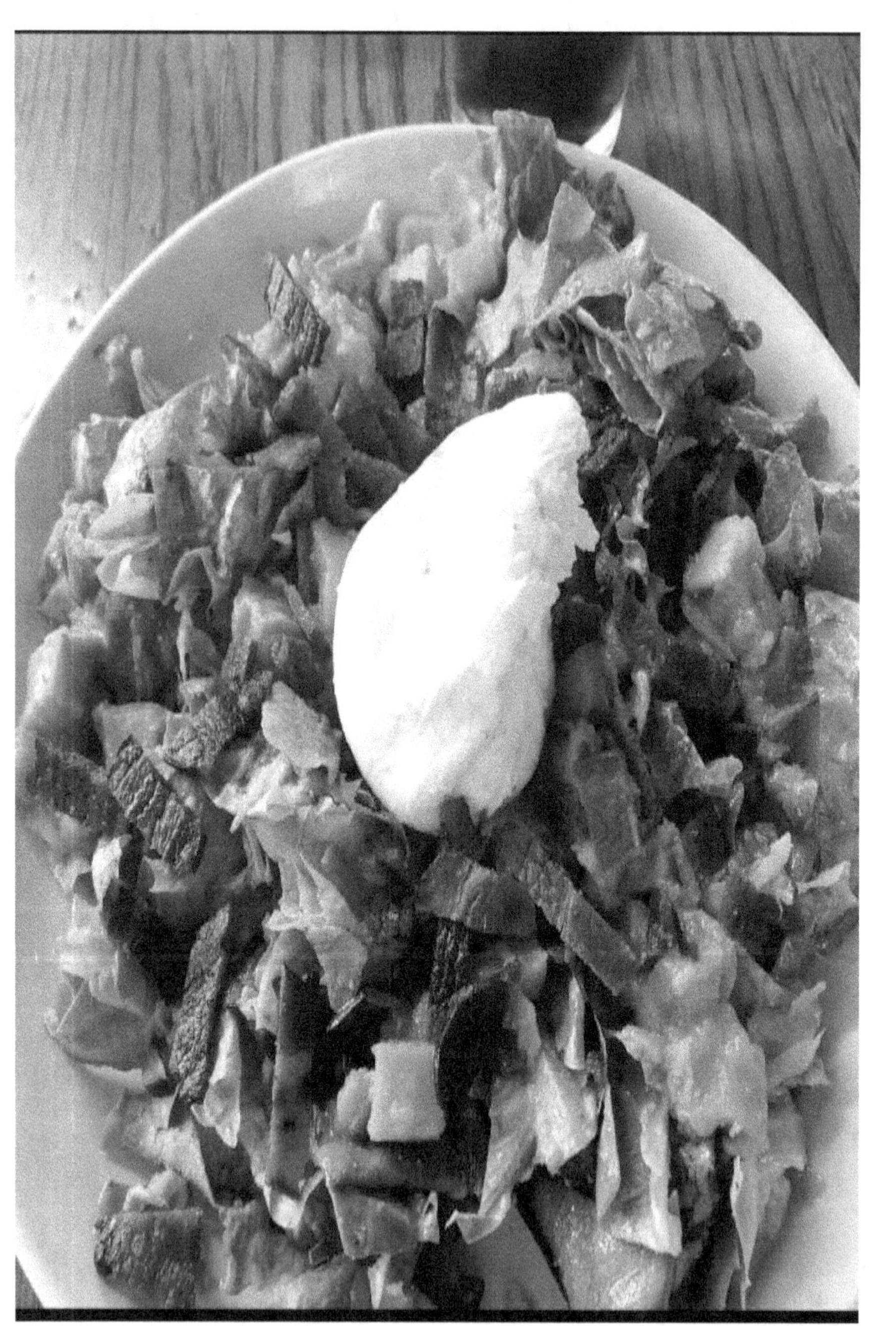

CHAPTER 6: 14-DAY MEAL PLAN FOR CKD STAGE 3 AND DIABETES TYPE 2

Day 1:

- Breakfast: Almond and Flaxseed Porridge (Recipe 1)
- Snack: Cucumber and Mint Yogurt Dip with vegetable sticks (Recipe 34)
- Lunch: Turkey and Vegetable Stuffed Peppers (Recipe 22)
- Snack: Baked Kale Chips with Nutritional Yeast (Recipe 31)
- Dinner: Lemon Herb Grilled Trout with a side of Grilled Asparagus with Lemon Zest (Recipe 21, Recipe 36)

Day 2:

- Breakfast: Greek Yogurt with Mixed Berries and Nuts (Recipe 3)
- Snack: Spiced Roasted Almonds (Recipe 35)
- Lunch: Spinach and Strawberry Salad with Balsamic Vinaigrette (Recipe 14)
- Snack: Celery Sticks with Almond Butter (Recipe 40)
- Dinner: Garlic and Herb Roasted Chicken Thighs with Garlic and Thyme Roasted Carrots (Recipe 24, Recipe 33)

Day 3:

- Breakfast: Egg White and Avocado Wrap (Recipe 5)
- Snack: Edamame Salad with Cherry Tomatoes (Recipe 37)
- Lunch: Asian Chicken Salad with Ginger Sesame Dressing (Recipe 17)
- Snack: Coconut Chia Seed Pudding (Recipe 44)
- Dinner: Zucchini Lasagna (Recipe 27)

Day 4:

- Breakfast: Oat Bran Pancakes with Blueberries (Recipe 10)
- Snack: Avocado and Black Bean Dip with whole-grain crackers (Recipe 38)
- Lunch: Arugula and Walnut Salad with Grilled Chicken (Recipe 13)
- Snack: Grilled Pineapple with Cinnamon Honey Drizzle (Recipe 45)
- Dinner: Quinoa Stuffed Portobello Mushrooms (Recipe 25)

Day 5:

- Breakfast: Low-Glycemic Muesli with Almonds (Recipe 6)
- Snack: Raspberry and Almond Flour Muffins (Recipe 42)
- Lunch: Watermelon and Feta Salad (Recipe 18)
- Snack: No-Bake Peanut Butter and Oat Bars (Recipe 47)
- Dinner: Shrimp and Cauliflower Grits (Recipe 26)

Day 6:

- Breakfast: Broccoli and Cheese Mini Quiches (Recipe 7)
- Snack: Dark Chocolate Avocado Truffles (Recipe 43)
- Lunch: Cucumber and Radish Salad with Dill Yogurt Dressing (Recipe 20)
- Snack: Baked Pears with Cinnamon and Walnuts (Recipe 41)
- Dinner: Moroccan Spiced Lamb Chops with a side of Green Bean and Almond Salad (Recipe 28, Recipe 39)

Day 7:

- Breakfast: Chia and Pumpkin Seed Pudding (Recipe 8)
- Snack: Kiwi and Lime Frozen Yogurt (Recipe 48)
- Lunch: Tomato and Avocado Gazpacho (Recipe 19)
- Snack: Strawberry and Basil Salad with Balsamic Reduction (Recipe 50)
- Dinner: Grilled Tilapia with Mango Salsa (Recipe 29)

Day 8:

- Breakfast: Spinach and Feta Breakfast Scramble (Recipe 2)
- Snack: Raspberry and Almond Flour Muffins (Recipe 42)
- Lunch: Zucchini Noodle Salad with Lemon Herb Dressing (Recipe 15)
- Snack: Baked Kale Chips with Nutritional Yeast (Recipe 31)
- Dinner: Baked Eggplant Parmesan (Recipe 23)

Day 9:

- Breakfast: Chia and Pumpkin Seed Pudding (Recipe 8)

- Snack: Spiced Roasted Almonds (Recipe 35)

- Lunch: Edamame Salad with Cherry Tomatoes (Recipe 37)

- Snack: Celery Sticks with Almond Butter (Recipe 40)

- Dinner: Garlic and Herb Roasted Chicken Thighs with Roasted Brussels Sprouts with Balsamic Glaze (Recipe 24, Recipe 32)

Day 10:

- Breakfast: Greek Yogurt with Mixed Berries and Nuts (Recipe 3)

- Snack: Avocado and Black Bean Dip with vegetable sticks (Recipe 38)

- Lunch: Arugula and Walnut Salad with Grilled Chicken (Recipe 13)

- Snack: Coconut Chia Seed Pudding (Recipe 44)

- Dinner: Lemon Herb Grilled Trout with a side of Grilled Asparagus with Lemon Zest (Recipe 21, Recipe 36)

Day 11:

- Breakfast: Low-Glycemic Muesli with Almonds (Recipe 6)

- Snack: Dark Chocolate Avocado Truffles (Recipe 43)

- Lunch: Watermelon and Feta Salad (Recipe 18)

- Snack: No-Bake Peanut Butter and Oat Bars (Recipe 47)

- Dinner: Quinoa Stuffed Portobello Mushrooms (Recipe 25)

Day 12:

- Breakfast: Broccoli and Cheese Mini Quiches (Recipe 7)

- Snack: Kiwi and Lime Frozen Yogurt (Recipe 48)

- Lunch: Tomato and Avocado Gazpacho (Recipe 19)

- Snack: Strawberry and Basil Salad with Balsamic Reduction (Recipe 50)

- Dinner: Shrimp and Cauliflower Grits (Recipe 26)

Day 13:

- Breakfast: Egg White and Avocado Wrap (Recipe 5)

- Snack: Grilled Pineapple with Cinnamon Honey Drizzle (Recipe 45)

- Lunch: Cucumber and Radish Salad with Dill Yogurt Dressing (Recipe 20)

- Snack: Baked Pears with Cinnamon and Walnuts (Recipe 41)
- Dinner: Moroccan Spiced Lamb Chops with a side of Green Bean and Almond Salad (Recipe 28, Recipe 39)

Day 14:

- Breakfast: Oat Bran Pancakes with Blueberries (Recipe 10)
- Snack: Raspberry and Almond Flour Muffins (Recipe 42)
- Lunch: Asian Chicken Salad with Ginger Sesame Dressing (Recipe 17)
- Snack: Avocado and Black Bean Dip with whole-grain crackers (Recipe 38)
- Dinner: Grilled Tilapia with Mango Salsa (Recipe 29)

Feel free to adjust the meal plan based on your personal preferences and nutritional needs. Remember to stay hydrated and consult with your healthcare provider or a registered dietitian to ensure that this meal plan is suitable for your specific health conditions.

Final Thoughts and Tips for Success:

As you embark on your journey to manage Chronic Kidney Disease (CKD) Stage 3 and Diabetes Type 2 through nutrition, remember that your diet plays a crucial role in your overall health and well-being. The recipes and meal plan provided in this cookbook are designed to support your dietary needs while offering delicious and satisfying options.

Here are some tips for success:

- ***Stay Hydrated:*** Drink plenty of water throughout the day to support kidney function and overall health.

- ***Monitor Portions:*** Be mindful of portion sizes to help manage blood sugar levels and maintain a healthy weight.

- ***Choose Whole Foods:*** Focus on whole, unprocessed foods to maximize nutrient intake and minimize additives and preservatives.

- ***Be Consistent:*** Consistency in your eating habits can help stabilize blood sugar levels and support kidney health.

- ***Listen to Your Body:*** Pay attention to how different foods affect your body and make adjustments as needed.

- ***Consult Professionals:*** Work closely with your healthcare team, including your doctor and dietitian, to tailor your diet to your specific needs.

Encouragement for Continued Health and Well-being:

Managing CKD Stage 3 and Diabetes Type 2 can be challenging, but with the right tools and mindset, you can lead a healthy and fulfilling life. Use this cookbook as a guide to inspire your culinary journey and support your dietary goals.

Remember that every step you take towards healthier eating habits is a positive move towards better health. Celebrate your successes, learn from your experiences, and stay motivated on your path to wellness.

We encourage you to continue exploring new recipes, experimenting with different flavors, and enjoying the process of cooking and eating nutritious meals. Your health is worth every effort, and we believe in your ability to succeed in managing your conditions through mindful nutrition and lifestyle choices.

Stay positive, stay committed, and embrace the journey to a healthier you!

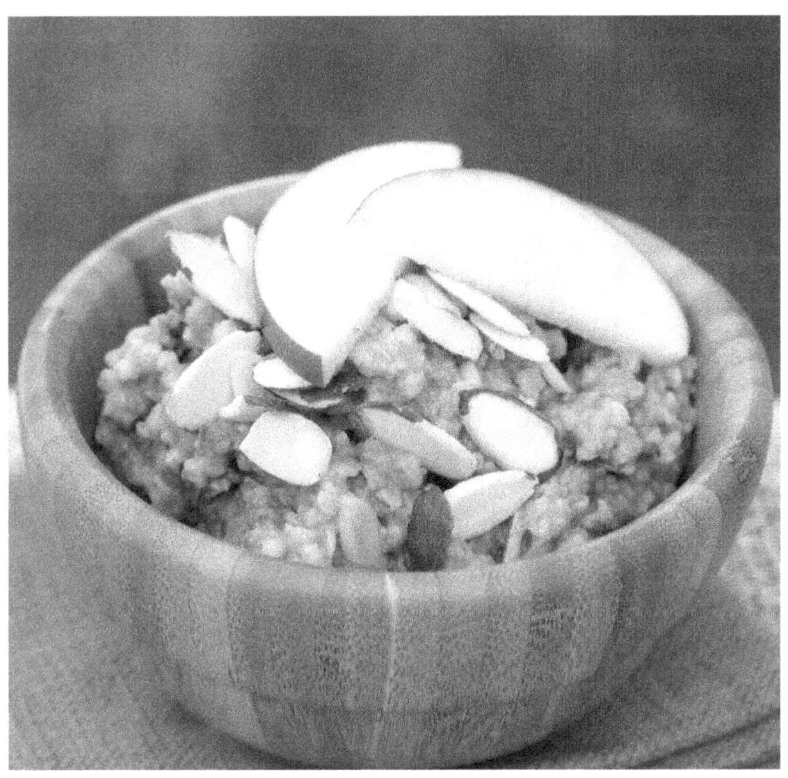

www.ingramcontent.com/pod-product-compliance
Lightning Source LLC
Chambersburg PA
CBHW070806260726

48660CB00005B/1733